Rheumatology

Efim Benenson

Rheumatology

Symptoms and Syndromes

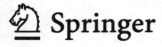
Springer

Author
Efim Benenson, MD
Professor of Medicine
Department of Internal Medicine
University of Cologne
Germany

The work was first published as a part of a work published in 2009 by Shaker Media in German laquage with the following title:

Rheumatologie: Syndrome and Algorithmen

Translation: Beverley Taylor

ISBN: 978-1-84996-461-6   e-ISBN: 978-1-84996-462-3
DOI: 10.1007/978-1-84996-462-3
Springer Dordrecht London Heidelberg New York

British Library Cataloguing in Publication Data
A catalogue record for this book is available from the British Library

Library of Congress Control Number: 2010936498

Cover design: eStudioCalamar, Figueres/Berlin

Printed on acid-free paper

Springer is part of Springer Science+Business Media (www.springer.com)

I dedicate this book to my wife, Irina, for her patience and support, our children, Anna and Vladimir, and to our grandchildren, Patrick, Paulina, and Wlada

Preface

"Symptoms and Syndromes" is aimed at teachers who are providing their trainees with further education and instruction in the relevant areas of clinical practice.

Features of the book:

- The classic textbook content of rheumatology is presented in the form of syndromes (or signs), as stable combinations of symptoms and usually with morphological and pathophysiological backgrounds, building a bridge or link between symptoms and diseases
- The principle of syndrome diagnosis which, in addition to the indispensable *description* of entities, should be integrated into the initial stages of clinical practice
- How to approach and structurally classify diseases from the viewpoint of morphological manifestations, as a fast route to diagnosis
- The clinical work from patient to disease, enabling preclinical and clinical knowledge on the concrete clinical case to be interlinked and stored in the long-term memory
- Algorithms of clinical reasoning, *leading to integrated staged diagnostics* based on morphology and pathophysiology
- A basic program of rheumatology comprising all teaching points (symptoms, syndromes, and diseases) linked to morphological structures, and connecting them to all clinical disciplines according to the broadly recognized terms of rheumatic diseases (see Contents)
- Inclusion of therapeutic and prognostic aspects of inflammatory arthritides, also touching on current therapeutic strategies and integrating them into the treatment concepts.

Practice-oriented clinical tuition (from syndromes and algorithms to diseases) is provided as a supplement to traditional descriptive teaching theory (from symptoms or disease pattern to diagnosis). On the one hand the book provides summaries of the most important clinical, imaging, and immunological syndromes as modules of rheumatology, while at the same time describing the medical approach to structured thinking, as an important tool for clinical practice. Such an approach enables the diversity of patients with rheumatic diseases to be clearly structured and categorized diagnostically.

The structure of the book reflects the said distinguishing features of other rheumatology books, providing fundamental information on the symptoms, signs, and therapeutic aspects of the diseases described therein. The Contents, in which all syndromes are easy to find and are linked to morphological structures, is both a manual and list of contents for this book.

Symptoms and Syndromes provides case-specific syndromes based on morphology and pathophysiology (Section 1, Articular and Musculoskeletal Disorders, Chapter 1-4 and Section 2, Connective Tissue Disease and Vasculitis, Chapter 8-10; Chapter 5 presents the paraneoplastic syndromes in rheumatology). These syndromes are linked in the text to specific diagnoses and represent a wide spectrum of differential diagnostics in internal medicine and its related fields. The approach relies on (auto) immunological phenomena and serological diagnostics (Chapter 11), and treatment-induced and associated conditions and diseases (Chapter 12) with a case-by-case study.

The algorithms and integrated staged diagnostics, using examples from Articular and Musculoskeletal Disorders (Chaps. 6 and 7), as well as Connective Tissue Diseases and Vasculitis (Chaps. 13 and 14), describe how the patient's information is to be analyzed. Actual therapeutic aspects of inflammatory rheumatic diseases are provided as examples in Chaps. 7.3 and Chaps 14.1–14.3.

This textbook is a reference work on the symptoms and syndromes of rheumatic diseases. It complements *Rheumatology: Clinical Scenarios* (E. Benenson, Springer 2011) with its 73 clinical situations and 164 illustrations, wherein all syndromes and symptoms from this collection are discussed with many other examples from my own practice as teaching modules in several chapters of *Symptoms and Syndromes*.

This stimulating concept combines *Symptoms and Syndromes* with *Clinical Scenarios* as case-based training, complementing one another in the same way as knowledge and its application, offering teachers an alternative training concept for trainees.

The book takes an alternative approach to rheumatic diseases. Thus it can help to reduce the time an experienced rheumatologist and physician requires for making a diagnostic decision, by applying structured knowledge, the syndrome principle of diagnosis and learning "to think clinically." By this means traditional teaching – from knowledge about diseases to the patient – is complemented. The critical comments on this book are really welcome (efim@benenson-rheumatologie.de).

Efim Benenson

Acknowledgments

Sincere thanks to my colleagues Professor of Medicine Michael Hallek, Director of Department I of Internal Medicine, University of Cologne for his advice and support, and my former boss, Professor of Medicine Volker Diehl, for welcoming me kindly to this Clinic in 1994, and especially Ursula Voigt-Pfeil for her active support in realizing this project.

Contents

Abbreviations

Ab	antibodies
ACE	angiotensin-converting enzyme
ACLA	anticardiolipin (antiphospholipid) antibody
ACR	American College of Rheumatology
ANA	antinuclear antibody
ANCA	anti-neutrophil cytoplasmic antibodies
APS	antiphospholipid syndrome
AS	ankylosing spondylitis
BASDAI	Bath Ankylosing Spondylitis Indices of Disease Activity
BVAS	Birmingham Vasculitis Activity Score
cANCA	cytoplasmic anti-neutrophil cytoplasmic antibody
Chap.	Chapter
CAPS	cryopyrin-associated periodic syndromes
C3, C4	components of the complement system
CCP	cyclic citrullinated peptide
CK	creatine kinase
CK-MB	isoenzyme of CK
CREST	calcinosis, Raynaud's phenomenon, esophageal dysmotility, sclerodactyly, teleangiectasia
CRMO	chronic recurrent multifocal osteomyelitis
CNS	central nervous system
COLD	chronic obstructive lung disease
CRP	C-reactive protein
Cry-V	cryoglobuline-associated vasculitis
CS	clinical situation
CSS	Churg-Strauss Syndrome
CT	computed tomography
CTD	connective tissue disease
CYC	cyclophosphamide
DAS	disease activity score
DD	differential diagnosis
DEXA	dual-energy X-ray absorptiometry

DIP	distal interphalangeal
DLCO	diffusing capacity for carbon monoxide
DM	dermatomyositis
DMARD	disease-modifying antirheumatic drug
dsDNA	double-stranded DNA
ssDNA	single-stranded DNA
ENA	extractable nuclear antigen
ENT	ear, nose and throat
ESR	erythrocyte sedimentation rate
FEV1	forced vital capacity in 1 sec
Fig.	figure
GGT	gamma glutamyl transferase
GOT	serum glutamic oxaloacetic transaminase
GPT	serum glutamic pyruvic transaminase
HAP	high-dose azathioprine pulse
HCV	hepatitis C virus
HBsAg	hepatitis B surface antigen
HIV	human immunodeficiexvncy virus
HLA-B27	human leukocyte antigen
HSV	hypersensitivity vasculitis
JIA	juvenile idiopathic arthritis
Ig	immunoglobulin
IL	interleukin
IM	intramuscular
IMIED	immune-mediated inner ear disease
IV	intravenous
Jo-1/Mi-2	myositis-specific antibody (designation of ENA antigens)
LDH	lactate dehydrogenase
LE	lupus erythematosus
MCP	metacarpophalangeal
MCTD	mixed connective tissue disease
MMF	mycophenolate mofetil
MPA	microscopic polyangiitis
MRI	magnetic resonance imaging
MS	multiple sclerosis
MTP	metatarsophalangeal
MTX	methotrexate
NHL	non-Hodgkin's lymphoma
NSAID	non-steroidal anti-inflammatory drug
OA	Osteoarthritis
OR	odds ratio relative risk
PAH	Pulmonary arterial hypertension
PAN	polyarteritis nodosa
p-ANCA	perinuclear anti-neutrophil cytoplasmic antibody
PCP	pneumocystis carinii pneumonia

PET	positron emission tomography
PHS	periarthropathy humeroscapularis
PIP	proximal interphalangial
PM/DM	polymyositis/dermatomyositis
PNS	paraneoplastic syndrome
PsA	psoriatic arthritis
RA	rheumatoid arthritis
RCS	Rheumatology: Clinical Scenarios (E. Benenson, Springer 2011)
ReA	reactive arthritis
RF	rheumatoid factor
RNP	ribonucleoprotein
RSO	radiosynoviorthesis
SAPHO	synovitis, acne, pustulosis, hyperostosis and osteitis
SC	subcutaneous
Scl-70	designation of specific ENA antigens (Topoisomerase-I)
SLEDAI	systemic lupus erythematosus disease activity index
SLE	systemic lupus erythematosus
SLICC	Systemic Lupus International Collaborating Clinics
Sm	Smith antigen
SpA	spondyloarthropathy
SSc	systemic sclerosis
SS-A (Ro)	designation of specific ENA antigens
SS-B (La)	designation of specific ENA antigens
STR	soft tissue rheumatism
TA	Takayasu arteritis
TB	tuberculosis
TNF	tumor necrosis factor
TSH	thyroid-stimulating hormone
VAS	visual analog scale
VDI	vasculitis damage index
WG	Wegener's granulomatosis

Articular and Musculoskeletal Disorder

This independent area of rheumatology is concerned primarily with clinical problems in the musculoskeletal system and is dealt with by rheumatologists and orthopedic specialists. Once the predominant medical and socioeconomic significance of these diseases has been illustrated, we can embark on the ideal journey toward diagnosis in arthrology. To this aim it is important to understand both the building blocks (lead symptoms and syndromes) as well as the mental algorithms.

Lead Symptoms and Syndromes

In the field of articular disorders /arthrology – just as in other clinical disciplines – there are general specialized terms and ultimately specific symptoms (lead symptoms) and syndromes.[1, 9, 10, 26] Lead symptoms set a precedent when it comes to diagnosis. Syndromes are the building blocks or foundation of diagnosis and can be ascertained from the morphological, pathophysiological, and clinical features of a disease. This becomes evident from Rheumatology Tree 1 presented on *Rheumatology: Clinical Scenarios* (E. Benenson, Springer 2011)-*RCS*, Chap. 1.3. The clinical data you have already collected (documentation of history and examinations, which should adequately guarantee the accuracy of the primary clinical data) are to be regarded as the fundamental premise for identifying the syndrome(s).

Articular Disorders

1

1.1
Arthralgia

This leading universal symptom in rheumatology is particularly important for achieving further differentiation[10, 14, 15]. Joint pain is often described as such if a pathomorphological substrate cannot be objectified and no external signs of inflammation (i.e., no tenderness) can be found. When considered in terms of morphology and pathophysiology, *arthralgia* may have not only articular, but also periarticular (Figs. 7[1], 128c, CS 53), osseous (Chaps. 3.10–3.11, Fig. 54), vascular (CS 71), functional and psychosomatic (Chap. 3.5, CS 57, 59, 61), or metabolic (*Fabry's* disease) origins.

Commonly occurring arthralgias have underlying functional and psychosomatic causes and the following pattern:

- Mostly in women, mono-/oligoarticular (hands, feet)
- Unstable, short-term, varying intensity
- Not movement induced, accompanied by vasospastic reactions
- Improvement after intake of sedatives

Such a pattern, of a highly psychosomatic nature, is also seen with *back pain* (cervicalgia, dorsalgia, and lumbalgia), chest pain (*thoracodynia*), and pain in the Achilles tendon (*achillodynia*). The diagnoses of such syndromes should be regarded as exclusion diagnoses, that is, they should only be made if all (and definitely all) organ-related diseases involving the same symptoms have been ruled out. This also applies, incidentally, to diffuse joint and muscular pain, which cannot be defined morphologically and is identified as *fibromyalgia*, *generalized tendomyopathy*, or a *global pain syndrome* (Chap. 3.5). Among the entire population, roughly three quarters of all chronic pain syndromes are caused by a disease of the musculoskeletal system (German Society of Rheumatology/DGRh/Healthcare Commission, June 2008, available on the Web). Such symptoms, which cannot be clearly defined, have recently been adopted as the diagnosis "pain disorder with somatic and psychological factors" in *ICD*-10 (*International Classification of Diseases*) under "somatoform disorders."

---

[1]All Fig./Figures/and clinical situations/CS/ are shown in "*Rheumatology: Clinical Scenarios*"/ *RCS*/ (E. Benenson, Springer 2011)

E. Benenson, *Rheumatology*, Symptoms and Syndromes
DOI: 10.1007/978-1-84996-462-3_1, © Springer-Verlag London Limited 2011

Fibromyalgic and inflammatory (see below) *arthralgias* are almost impossible to differentiate in one patient. For this reason, more recent *RA* studies ask patients to complete two specific questionnaires aimed selectively at *RA* and *fibromyalgia*. Patients with high grade *fibromyalgia* should not be classified in the *RA* studies on account of the difficulties with assessing efficacy described below.

Otherwise, patients with *arthralgias* and other local or diffuse pain symptoms who usually can be denoted as having "non-rheumatic" diseases, should initially be cared for by their general practitioner and do not necessarily require primary rheumatological investigation.

The demarcations between inflammatory and noninflammatory *arthralgias* can also be regarded as a problem in everyday rheumatology, which cannot always be solved. This applies in particular if there is an inflammatory disease, where the main question is the type of pain which predominates.

This is illustrated by CS 57, for example, wherein a male patient with *PsA* but minimal activity had severe polyarthralgias with restricted movement in the hands. As a result he was placed on sick leave for a number of months and ultimately was discharged from cure therapy due to an attack of his underlying disease. This could not be confirmed by subsequent examinations, however. The Remicade® therapy (three infusions), applied with the aim of differentiating between inflammatory and noninflammatory pain, had little effect.

The same difficulties with differentiation can be seen in CS 59 and 61.

Stable *arthralgias* with a specific pattern over a certain time period have greater clinical relevance if they are of an "inflammatory" and "mechanical" nature. Such arthralgias should at least undergo rheumatological or orthopedic investigation. In such an event there could be a nasty surprise waiting, as in the case of Fig. 54, where a bone tumor was ultimately identified in the presence of severe arthralgia (with later swelling), and postoperatively as a *stress fracture*, or in the case of one of our female patients, aged 42, in whom massive *polyarthralgia* preceded *retrobulbar granuloma*, as shown in Fig. 96. Arthralgia of the temporomandibular joint causes local pain, which may extend to the face and head.

"Inflammatory" *arthralgias* (articular and periarticular) have the following features:

- Oligo-/polyarticular
- Stable, intensive, and long-term (up to 24 h) pain
- Mostly nocturnal, early morning
- Morning stiffness
- Improvement on exercise

Such *arthralgias* must mostly be ascribed to *arthritis*.

"Mechanical" *arthralgias* are characterized as follows:

- Mono-/oligoarticular, large or small joints, not intensive to begin with
- Pain after static and mechanical strain
- Pain mostly on initial movement (run-in pain) and in the evenings
- Improvement with rest

Such a pattern of arthralgia is very closely linked to the initial stage of degenerative joint disease (*osteoarthritis [OA]*) or spinal disease (*osteochondrosis*).

When both patterns are combined and the severity of the muscular pain, the adaptive posture and restricted movements are not proportionately related to the conventional clinical picture, an osseous cause should be considered – namely, *aseptic bone necroses* (Chap. 9.9, CS 44) or *stress fracture* (Fig. 54); more extensive, appropriate imaging procedures (bone scintigraphy, MRI) should be undertaken. Most frequently, idiopathic necroses of the femoral head (*Perthes* disease) or other causes and localizations (e.g., knee – primary or secondary *Ahlbäck's* disease, tarsal bone – *Schlatter's* disease, carpal bone – *Köhler's* disease) are involved. *Aseptic necroses* gain in importance during intensive cortisone therapy and immunosuppression, often in *RA or ReA* (CS 44, Fig. 121), *SLE* or patients with a kidney or liver transplant.

1.2
Morning Stiffness

This lead symptom is characterized by non-painful, restricted movement and diminished well-being, especially on initial movement, though it abates after a while. The same difficulties occur after periods of rest. Such a symptom is measured by its intensity and duration and is indicative of the activity of joint disease. If it lasts more than 1 h before maximal improvement, such a symptom has nosological specificity for *RA* (a primary and first diagnostic criterion) and for *Polymyalgia rheumatica,* if it lasts for any more than 45 min.

1.3
Arthritis

This is the most common syndrome and most frequent admission diagnosis in rheumatology! It involves an inflammation of the synovial membrane (*synovialitis*). A differentiation is made between *primary* and *secondary arthritis.* Synovialitis in *primary arthritis* could, depending on evaluation, cause cartilage and bone destruction as a result of pannus formation. Consequently, secondary *OA* develops (Chap. 1.4). *Secondary arthritis*, which is mainly associated with *OA*, entails the irritation of the synovial membrane.

The clinical diagnosis of *inflammatory arthritis* is justified by:

- The "*inflammatory*" nature of the *arthralgias* (see above) and the following symptoms:
- Tenderness (scored by the patient on the VAS from one to three points)
- Synovialitic (in contrast to the cases in which the periarticular structures are primarily affected, Figs. 7, 128c) swelling (judged by the physician on the scale of 1–3 points)
- Restrictions to active movement (painful movement deficits)

The clinical severity, rating, and advancement of the *arthritis* vary, irrespective of the pathomorphological changes which predominate in the joints at the given time. The most common forms of *arthritis* have their own designations: *gonarthritis* (knee), *omarthritis* (shoulder), *coxarthritis* (hip). A distinction is made between the following types of arthritis (in the subsequent figure you should recognize the changes described below):

1.3.1
Exudative (Inflammatory) Arthritis

Exudative arthritis (Figs. 3, 13, 21, 24, 25, 40, 41, 49a, 68, 115, 128a, 129a) indicates the *florid,* highly active form of *arthritis* and is manifested as:

- Swelling of periarticular structures (up to three points on the scale), often with spindle-shaped finger joints, possibly from the erythema or reddening (Fig. 13)
- Palpable warmth of the joint
- Palpable effusions in the joint
- Joint tenderness (up to three points on the VAS, 0–3)
- Painful limitation to active movement

Such forms of *arthritis* are indicators of (sub) *acute rheumatic disease* or an episode of such diseases (*RA, ReA, PsA, SpA, podagra* in *gout arthritis, pseudogout* as a polyarticular form) or of others, for example, in association with microbial (Yersinia, rheumatic fever, borreliosis, Gonococci, TB, sepsis) and viral (hepatitis B, C, HIV, parvovirus B19) infections or with *hyperlipidemia.* At the same time, other conditions (e.g., *osteoarthritis* with *synovitis, algodystrophy* stages I, *aseptic necroses)* and above all *bone tumor* or *stress fracture* (Fig. 54) should be taken into consideration. Forms of arthritis in *Löfgren's* syndrome with *sarcoidosis* in fact signify acute *periarthritis,* since histologically there is no synovialitis. When excluding such a disease, other rare causes for the swollen joints are feasible, namely, *hydrops intermittens, villonodular synovitis* (knee involvement is typical to both), *palindromic rheumatism.*

1.3.2
Proliferative Arthritis

Proliferative arthritis (Figs. 5, 35, 58, 80, 104, 129c) is to be regarded primarily as a spontaneous or drug-induced regression of exudative synovialitis or its progression to *pannus formation,* and is manifested as:

- *Arthralgia* only upon movement, seldom at rest
- Hardening of periarticular structures, swelling (1–2 points)
- Infiltration of exudate in the bursae (hard *bursitis*)
- *Amyotrophies* (atrophy of *Mm. interossei*), specific to *RA* (unlike *osteoarthritis* or diseases with asymmetric involvement of the finger joints)
- *Disfiguration*: transformation of the joint surface as a result of exudative and proliferative changes to the joints (effusions) and periarticular structures (swelling)
- *Deformity*: transformation of the joint surface(s) as a result of changes to the bone structures of the joint

- Minimal tenderness (VAS 1–2 points)
- Painful (active) and non-painful (passive) movement deficits

1.3.3
Fibrosing and Ankylosing Arthritis

Fibrosing and ankylosing arthritis (Figs. 5, 35, 42, 43, 62, 80, 104, 129c) possibly an indication of antecedent synovial inflammation, is viewed as a latent sequela of exudative-proliferative inflammation, pannus formation, and cartilage and bone destruction in *RA, PsA*, chronic *gout arthritis, algodystrophy* stage III. Such joint changes are manifested as:

- Minimal *arthralgias*, tenderness, and swelling.
- *Contractures* (osseous adhesions or adhesions of different layers of the periarticular structures, namely, the skin, fasciae, tendon sheaths, muscles, Figs. 5, 40, 43, 63, 70, 80, 95, 104, 129c); when extreme, known as *claw hand, arthrogenic* (Fig. 62 in *RA*, Fig. 130a in *OA*), *dermatogenic* (Fig. 18), or *neurogenic* (Fig. 19).
- *Disfiguration* (due to synovitis, *bursitis*, and *tenosynovitis* of the extensor tendons, Figs. 3, 13, 15a, 21, 28, 40, 42, 49a, 58, 65a, 68, 104, 115, 129a). Following effective therapy, disfiguration is mostly reversible (Fig. 15b). DD with *puffy hands* (Figs. 7, 66) and periarticular swelling (Fig. 128c).
- *Deformity*: buttonhole (Fig. 62, DD in *OA*, Fig. 81), swan-neck (Fig. 5, Dig. 3 left), *Jaccoud's* arthropathy with *CTD* (*MCTD*, Fig. 70: only the tendons and ligaments affected here), DD with finger *OA* (Figs. 4, 128a).
- *Ankylosis* (osseous adhesions or surgical fusion/stiffening/of the joints)/Figs. 9a, 42, 43, 51, 62; also after arthrodesis, Figs. 104 and 122c/.
- *Deviations* – lateral (ulnar) deviations of the wrists and fingers (Figs. 42, 43, 70).
- *Mutilations*, spontaneous osteolysis (Fig. 42, digit 1 left, 4–5 bilaterally, Fig. 104, Dig. 5 on both sides) described as *Arthritis mutilans*, and in *PsA* as *"pencil-in-cup."*
- *(Sub) luxations* (partial or full incongruence or dislocation of the joint surfaces, most commonly in the MCP joints) leading to chronic painful functional impairment (Figs. 5, 9, 42, 43, 59, 62 right , 104).

1.3.4
Erosive Arthritis

The *bone destruction* is diagnosed by imaging, namely, by X-ray *morphology* (Figs. 9a, 51, 59, 119), CT (Figs. 23, 34, 45), or MRI (Figs. 122ab). Such changes in morphology are closely associated with the osteoclast activity and pannus formation typical of these specific diseases and are indicative of the features of chronic *synovitis* in *RA, PsA* and other forms of *SpA,* as well as the other causes of bone destruction (*gout arthritis, septic arthritis*/late stages/, *Still's* disease (in up to 50% of all cases), *familial Mediterranean fever*/knee-hip/, seldom *SLE, algodystrophy* stage II). Figure 34 depicts destruction in a number of bones and *osteolyses* (refer to the comments on this case in *RCS*, Chap. 2).

The bone destruction is consistent only with certain entities. In this regard, it is a discriminatory (between erosive and non-erosive joint diseases), diagnostic (a primary criterion of *RA* but also *PsA* and *gout arthritis*), and prognostic (the *severity* of the *RA* is defined by the stage, 0–4 according to *Steinbrocker*, →Chap. 6.8) sign. The erosions occur relatively early (e.g., during the first weeks and months of *RA*), and thus express the destructive potential of joint disease. Conversely, the absent or untypical (in terms of the pattern) erosive changes during the foreseeable period, possibly a few years (CS 2, 24 and 53), rule out certain diseases, for example, *RA, gout arthritis, PsA*, almost exclusively.

The potential erosive/destructive changes are essentially regarded as the major targets (together with the disease activity and functional disorders) for basic therapy of such diseases. Advanced joint destruction can also be found amongst the clinical syndromes (*deformities, bony ankylosis, mutilations*) → *RCS*, Chap. 1.3.3.

The varying degree and the combinations of such clinical, morphological, and radiological changes reflect, over the long term, the multifaceted symptoms of chronic joint disease (most often affecting *RA*, but also the other destructive forms of arthritis) and trophic effects on tissue damage (e.g., *algodystrophy* stage III).

1.3.5
Non-erosive Arthritis

Non-erosive arthritis (Fig. 72) in other rheumatic and non-rheumatic diseases are, predominantly, of essential importance to differential diagnosis (CS 2, 24 and 53), with a good prognosis in terms of the joints.

1.4
Osteoarthritis

This is the name for a mostly degenerative joint condition, whereby destruction of the cartilage results in chronic pain and functional impairment. *Primary (idiopathic) OA* is most common and widespread (with an incidence of almost 100% in those aged over 60), induced predominantly by mechanical factors and (over)exertion disproportionate to personal resilience. Initially, there are no signs of inflammation. *OA* is the most common cause of chronic noninflammatory polyarthritis though they do appear as the disease progresses. Such a condition is defined as *reactive synovitis* and should be regarded as an irritation of the synovial membrane or *secondary arthritis*. Therefore, a differentiation is made between two forms of *AO*: noninflammatory and inflammatory (with *synovitis*).

The distinction between inflammatory and noninflammatory processes is critical.

1.4.1
Noninflammatory OA

Noninflammatory OA is characterized by:

- The "mechanical" nature of *arthralgias* (see above)
- Run-in pain, pain on exercise and at rest in the joints, upon the greatest mechanical exertion possible

- Restricted *passive* (with a lack of ossification of the joints and accompanying *contractures*, Fig. 130a) movements, including *claw hand* (Fig. 62), *hammer toe* (Fig. 43), often sensitive *callosities* and *corns* (clavi) as a result (in the patients with *RA* stage IV)
- Hard tissue (bony) enlargements in the small joints: DIP (*Heberden's* nodes) and a similar process in the PIP (*Bouchard's* nodes) joints
- Marked crepitus on movement in the thumb base
- No tenderness
- No swelling

1.4.2
Inflammatory OA

Inflammatory OA is explained by:

- The above mentioned symptoms of noninflammatory *OA* plus some local inflammatory symptoms:
  - Increased, persistent, and intensive arthralgias
  - Tenderness, swelling, disfiguration
  - Painful, swollen, reddened *Heberden's* and *Bouchard's* nodes, and the *thumb base*
- Restricted active (due to pain) movements

In *OA*, such clinical problems concentrate primarily in certain joints, also by way of definition and on account of specific radiological changes (Chap. 6.8). Joint involvement in *OA* is usually focal rather than generalized. They have the following most common forms of *OA*:

- *Heberden's* nodes (distal finger interphalangeal joints)/Figs. 3, 4, and 8, X-ray for the same patient, 5, 42, 81, 89; 128b/.
- *Thumb base*/Figs. 9ab, 59/, osteophytes may lead to this "squared" appearance.
- *Bouchard's* nodes (proximal finger interphalangeal joints)/Figs. 4 and 8, X-ray for the same patient, 81, 128a; X-ray 128b/.
- *Hip*/Fig. 97/, often as congenital or developmental defects (e.g., acetabular dysplasia), bilateral involvement (in 20%), can present itself as knee pain.
- *Knee*/Fig. 26/may result in a *varus* (involvement of the medial compartment) or a *valgus* (lateral compartment) *deformity;* a "shrug" may be a sign of the patellofemoral joint or *chondromalacia* patellae.
- *Shoulder* and acromioclavicular joints.
- *Hallux rigidus* (first MTP)/Fig. 43/.
- *Spine*/Fig. 60 shows cervical spine, but with specific inflammatory signs of another disease – which?/(see Chap. 2.3).
- *Generalized OA* is characterized by involvement of three or more joints or groups of small joints (DIP und PIP joints are counted as one group each).
- The clinical severity of *OA* often correlates poorly with radiographic findings.

1.4.3
Secondary OA

Secondary OA appears pathologically indistinguishable from idiopathic *OA*, is known by the "*OA*-like" symptoms (e.g., pain without swelling) induced by chronic *arthritis* and other multiplicity causes. Such symptoms arise most often from:

- Other joint diseases (*RA*, septic *arthritis* → Chap. 1.3.3)
- Bone diseases (fracture, infection, *aseptic necrosis* → Chap. 3.10)
- Iatrogenic after intensified intra-articular therapy with cortisone, or after RSO and surgical synovectomy, respectively
- Trauma (acute, sports)
- Congenital or developmental (e.g., hip dislocation, bone dysplasias, unequal lower extremity length)
- *Arthropathies* (neuropathic, metabolic u.a), whereby the dystrophic changes are accompanied by inflammatory changes (Chap. 1.5)

In clinical terms, the intensive (more than previously) motion-dependent *arthralgias* predominate and are totally disproportionate to the current, minimal *exudative-proliferative arthritis*, as can be deduced from CS 35. At the same time, the arthrotic changes can be assessed through imaging techniques (X-ray, bone scan). Such a transformation in the clinical and imaging pattern is often seen in advanced stages of *destructive* "spent" *arthritis*.

1.4.4
Erosive OA

Erosive OA particularly of the finger joints is certainly the most prominently affected and most difficult problem to identify in arthrology. Erosive OA tends to be more destructive than typical *OA*. The diagnosis is first obtained clinically based on the *deformities* and *(sub) luxations* (Figs. 4, 81, CS 28) and radiologically (erosive changes and *osteolysis*, Fig. 8). If the involvement is isolated to the PIP joints (Figs. 4 and 128ab), which could be equally affected in *Bouchard's OA* and *RA* (cf. Figs. 8 and 9a), differentiation is particularly difficult, and all the more so if there are no specific markers for *RA*.

It is important here to consider the neighboring joints: MCP involvement is by no means typical of *OA*, but very typical of *RA* (Fig. 9b), whereas DIP joints are indicative explicitly of *Heberden's OA* (here there is – anatomically – no synovial membrane and *synovitis* therefore is not possible). *Erosive OA* (Figs. 4, 8, 81) cannot be easily distinguished from *erosive arthritis* (Chap. 1.3.4, Figs. 5, 9a, 129c). This applies in particular if *RA* arises from long-term *Bouchard's OA*. This, not uncommon concurrence of *OA* with *RA*, is known as *late-onset arthritis*. The important cause of *erosive OA*, if selective involvement of MCP 2–3 is the case (as shown in Figs. 58–59, 129a), is *hemochromatosis*

(Chap. 1.5.3). To differentiate here from *RA* it is important to document the overall joint status and especially the *pattern of involvement*, presenting as *OA* with *synovitis* and not as *RA*, as well as *ferritin* and *anti-CCP*-Ab, which in our case (CS 50), after long-term MTX therapy, certainly permits the correct pathogenetic treatment (blood-letting), without MTX, to be determined.

1.4.5
Chondrocalcinosis

Chondrocalcinosis takes the form of linear, partly patchy deposits in the cartilage (menisci) and also in the synovial membrane of calcium pyrophosphate dihydrate crystals with symptoms of *pseudogout* (Chap. 1.5.3), often in *hyperparathyroidism* (Chap. 1.5.2).

1.4.6
Chondromatosis

Chondromatosis is characterized by symptoms of (non)inflammatory *OA* and recurrent joint blocks (on account of the numerous chondromas formed in the synovial membrane and appearing as loose bodies in the intra-articular space). *Chondromalacia* is characterized clinically (Fig. 25) by mostly peripatellar pain in the knee (described as *patella* syndrome), and morphologically (Fig. 26) by defibration of the cartilage of the patella (CS 9).

1.4.7
Arthritis and Osteoarthritis

The term *osteoarthritis* (*OA*) is rightly used in English specialist terminology for emphasizing a pathogenetically important and to some extent common inflammatory component of *arthritis* and *OA*.

OA is now considered to be a systemic inflammatory condition that affects all components of the joint, including subchondral bone.

Clinically, it is important, due to the sometimes similar symptoms (pain, swelling, restricted mobility), to identify these two heterogeneous diseases as early as possible.

As a diagnosis, the term *OA-arthritis* carries a certain degree of uncertainty and could almost be seen as a makeshift response if essentially, it is not possible to distinguish between these two conditions.

In this respect, the following must be considered: how and in which order did the symptoms appear? If the pain occurs together with swelling, the initial thought should be systemic, inflammatory joint disease. If the pain, even of a mechanical nature, is not accompanied by swelling but this is possibly the case much later, such a constellation is more likely to be interpreted as *primary OA*, possibly with *secondary arthritis*.

The *pattern of involvement* is of great importance thereby:

- In the DIP joints it could only be *OA* with inflammatory (Figs. 3, 4, 8) or *PsA* (hot spots, Fig. 64).
- In the PIP joints there are manifestations of both *OA* with inflammatory (Figs. 4, 8, 81, 89, 128ab) and *arthritis* (Figs. 3, 5, 9a, 28, 35, 40, 49, 62, 64, 68, 80, 104, 129a).
- Involvement of the several small (MCP) and medium-large (wrist) joints (Figs. 5, 9ab, 21, 28, 35, 40, 42, 49ab, 80, 89, 104, 115, 129ac) is associated, almost exclusively, with *RA* and other inflammatory joint diseases, including parvovirus infection, or rarely *pseudogout*.

The term *OA-arthritis* is derived from the description of the radiological findings, wherein the signs of both conditions are seen but the *primary* articular disease is the aim of the radiological finding and should be defined thereby. Using the listed figure, you can sharpen your senses to *osteoarthritis-arthritis*.

1.5
Arthropathy

This comprehensive syndrome is described pathogenetically as *dystrophic* joint changes, which in causative terms have neurological, metabolic, endocrinological, and tumorous associations. Clinically, it is manifested as joint involvement in the various non-rheumatic diseases and presents as a complex, variable syndrome of *arthralgias*, *degenerative* (Chap. 1.4) and *inflammatory* (Chap. 1.3) symptoms. These include all conditions involving joint problems, which by definition can be attributed neither to *primary arthritis* (cf. Rheumatology Tree 1, *RCS*, Chap. 1.3) nor to *primary OA*.

This term is generally used in a broad sense, perhaps, not as the nosological diagnosis but to describe rheumatic syndromes associated with infections (infectious arthropathies) or with *primary* forms of *arthritis* (inflammatory polyarthropathies), as well as a preliminary diagnosis if, in *arthralgias* and *back pain*, inflammatory changes in the joints or the spine cannot be identified or ruled out. This is the case, for instance, with unconfirmed *SpA* or joint symptoms in *psoriasis* (talking now of *PsA*).

Problems with the joints in *arthropathies* are characterized by:

- *Arthralgias*
- A colorful combination of noninflammatory and inflammatory changes
- Concurrent symptoms within the context of soft-tissue rheumatism/*STR*/ (see below)

The most common *arthropathies* are associated with related diseases.

1.5.1
Neuropathic Arthropathy

(Synonyms: *"neurotrophic arthritis"*, *"Charcot's arthropathy" or joints*)

This is a severe form of *OA* associated with loss of pain sensation, proprioception, or both.
　　Types of joint changes:

- Mostly monoarticular
- Noninflammatory, pain-free joint involvement
  - Initially pain-free periarticular swelling, articular effusions
  - Later osteoporosis, joint and/or bone destruction with *deformations, luxations*

The most significant causes or diseases of the

- CNS:
  - *Syringomyelia, syphilis* (*Tabes dorsales*), *MS, tetraplegia* (Fig. 19)
  - *Massive destructive changes* in the large joints and *spine*
- *Peripheral nervous system:*
  - *Diabetes mellitus* with the following connective tissue symptoms:
    - *Diabetic hand* syndrome, *"stiff hand," "scleroderma-like syndrome"*
    - *"Fat fingers"* (Fig. 130a), *contractures* of the finger joints (Fig. 19) without acral necrosis
    - *Destructive arthritis* (osteolyses) in tarsal and ankle joints, described as diabetic flat foot, with mostly pain-free swelling, *subluxations, mutilations, and ankyloses* (due to osteopathic *osteonecroses*, concomitant *neuropathy* and tarsometatarsal joint destruction)
    - *Cheiroarthropathy* (limited joint mobility)
    - *Ankylosing hyperostosis* of the spine (*Forestier's* disease) with stiffness and typical radiological changes (Fig. 118), *osteoporosis*
    - *Dupuytren's* contracture (Fig. 95)
    - *Carpal tunnel* syndrome
    - *Rotator cuff disease* (capsulitis/tendinitis of the shoulder, as in Fig. 106)
    - *Foot ulceration*

"Charcot's arthropathy" occurs in 0.1–2.0% of patients with diabetes and is by far the most common disorder.

- *Neurodystrophy, primary* (idiopathic) and *secondary* (post-traumatic, neurological, rheumatic diseases, paraneoplastic). Synonyms: *algodystrophy*, reflex dystrophy syndrome, complex regional pain syndrome, *Sudeck's* disease:
  - *Acute mono-/oligoarthritis* and *periarthritis* (in foot/shoulder with severe pain, swelling, reddening, and extremely elevated *CRP*)

- *Proliferative (peri) arthritis* with cyanotic, hardened swelling, periarticular fibrosis, and joint stiffness, also pain and increased signs of inflammation
- *Atrophy* of *periarticular* structures and muscles, capsular shrinking, *contractures*

1.5.2
Endocrinological Arthropathy

- *Acromegaly:*
  - Degenerative *arthropathy* and *spondylopathy* with osteophyte formation
  - Cutaneous soft-tissue growth (hands and feet), periarticular calcifications
  - *Carpal tunnel* syndrome
  - *Myopathies* (myasthenia and myalgia)
- *Hyperparathyroidism* (*primary*/CS 67/and *secondary* in *sarcoidosis*, renal insufficiency, *neoplasias*/CS 56/, malabsorption):
  - Back and joint pain
  - *Osteoporosis* in the joints and spine
  - Erosion, osteolyses, and multiple cysts/as in Fig. 34/, periostal resorption, *chondrocalcinosis* (MCP, femur, tibia, sacroiliac joints)
  - *Myopathies* with myasthenia
  - *Enthesiopathies*
  - *Secondary* (from *(pseudo) gout* and soft-tissue calcifications)
  - (Peri) *arthritis*
  - *Elevated* serum levels of calcium, creatinine, uric acid, parathormone (remaining normal with *neoplasias*, CS 56), *and low phosphate*
- ❖ *Hypercalcemia* syndrome. Serum *calcium > 3.5 mmol/L* in non-clotted blood signifies an *emergency:*
  - Initially asymptomatic (CS 56, 67), requires emergency treatment
  - Followed by hypotension, vomiting, dehydration, abdominal pain, disorientation
- *Hypo-/hyperthyroidism*:
  - Swollen fingers, capsule thickening in *hypothyroidism*
  - *Myopathy* (mainly proximal) in *hyper-/hypothyroidism, myalgia* in *hypothyroidism* (CS 54)
  - *Enthesopathies* in hyperthyroidism

1.5.3
Metabolic Arthropathy

- *Crystallopathies*
  - *Gout arthritis* (*hyperuricemia* men *> 7.0–7.7 mg/dL*, women *> 6.0–6.5 mg/dL*, Figs. 13, 130b):
    - *Acute* (pain-free interval between episodes of gout, hyperuricemia in 90%):

❖ – Emergency symbol

- Highly acute arthritis in first metatarsophalangeal joint (*podagra*) or knee or much more rarely in other joints, such as PIP (Fig. 13)
- Fever, chills
- Triggers: excessively fatty food with alcohol, infection, surgery
- Serum urate levels are often normal during acute attacks especially in allopurinol users
- *Chronic* (*no pain-free interval*), persistent *polyarthritis* (CS 55)[18]:
  - Exudative and/or fibrosing, *destructive arthritis* with osseous tophi (Fig. 130b)
  - Extra-articular urate deposits: soft-tissue tophi in the hands, feet, auricles
- *Pseudogout arthritis* (*chondrocalcinosis*, *primary* and *secondary*, or calcium pyrophosphate dihydrate (CPPD) crystal deposition disease → Chap. 1.5.2):
  - *Acute* (ESR, CRP elevated, no hyperuricemia):
    - *Arthritis* (mostly *knee joint* and other large joints, hardly ever *podagra*)
    - Non-erosive changes to small joints, possibly erosions of large joints
  - *Chronic*:
    - Calcifications often of menisci (in the knee) and joint cartilage (triangular fibrocartilage of the wrist)/radiological findings/
    - *Secondary OA* with calcifications in menisci and hyaline cartilage
    - *Periarthropathy* (tenosynovitis) in the region of the shoulder and wrist
    - *Spondylopathy* (intervertebral discs, around the axis, of lower cervical and whole lumbar spine or in ligamentum flavum)
    - No visceral manifestations
    - Calcifications are high in the elderly patients but asymptomatic or subclinical in many cases
- *Hemochromatosis* (CS 50):
  - *Erosive arthritis* on account of *OA* with synovitis, explicitly in MCP 2–3 bilaterally (Figs. 58, 59, 129a)
  - *OA* and *chondrocalcinosis*, then
  - *Arthritis* of the large and small joints (due to deposits of iron and calcium pyrophosphate crystals with symptoms of *pseudogout*)
  - *Organ involvement*: liver, heart, gonads, skin
  - *Elevated serum iron, ferritin and transferrin* saturation, normal CRP and ESR levels

1.5.4
Hematological Arthropathy

- *Hemophilic arthropathy* or hemarthrosis (joint hemorrhage):
  - *Initial* acute *exudative arthritis* (Chap. 1.3.1) mostly of the large joints (knees, ankles, elbows, shoulders, DD *septic arthritis*) with hematoma and episodes of bleeding (intermittent course)

- *Proliferative, fibrosing-ankylosing arthritis* (Chap. 1.3.3) arising from more developed chronic synovialitis with pannus formation and subsequently *RA* and (*secondary*) *OA*-type, destructive joint changes, along with their sequelae (*contractures, ankyloses*)
- *Leukemic synovialitis*:
  - *Arthralgia* and *arthritis* (knees, ankles) in acute leukemia, rarely in chronic leukemia, DD *bone tumors* or *stress fracture* (Fig. 54)

1.5.5
Enteropathic Arthropathy

- *ReA* or *Yersinia* induced (Chap. 11.3.2, CS 37, 69; Fig. 102; CS 60)
  - *Oligoarthritis,* asymmetric, predominantly of lower extremities (knees)
  - *Tendinitis, enthesiopathies*
  - *Sacroiliitis,* unilateral or bilateral (as in Figs. 44–46)
- *Crohn's* disease and *ulcerative colitis* have the same connective tissue symptoms:
- *Whipple's* disease, chronic inflammation of the jejunum, induced by *Tropheryma whipplei*
  - Asymmetric *oligoarthritis*, subcutaneous *nodules, hyperpigmentation* of the skin
  - *Fever* (general health deteriorated), *malabsorption* (diarrhea), organ (heart, lungs, liver) involvement
  - Diagnosis confirmed by *small intestine biopsy* and response to *tetracycline* (such a response was seen in *borreliosis,* Figs. 20ab)

1.5.6
Paraneoplastic Arthropathy

(See Chap. 5)

- *Hypertrophic osteoarthropathy*:
  - *Arthralgia, myopathy*
  - *Drumstick fingers, hour-glass nails* (Fig. 88) also in *psoriasis* (as in this case, acute in HIV patient), *hyperthyroidism*

1.6
Extra-articular Organ Involvement

Extra-articular (systemic) symptoms, as a rule, represent a serious, highly complicated course of *arthritis* and arthropathy, could have underlying drug toxicity, and are suspected on account of:

- Polyarticular involvement and high-grade activity
- Proof of *rheumatoid nodules* (Chap. 3.1.1) and high-titer of *RF, anti-CCP*-Ab and *ANA* (Chap. 6.7)
- In such cases, an active investigation should ensue for involvement of:
  - Skin and subcutaneous tissue: *rheumatoid nodules* (Figs. 35, 80, 104, 122), *palmar erythema* (Fig. 100), deep *ulcerations* (Fig. 101a), cortisone-induced atrophy and scars (Fig. 101b)
  - Musculature (low-lying rheumatoid nodules/CS 45, Figs. 122ab, *amyotrophy, myositis,* corticoid myopathy)
  - Vessels (*vasculopathy, vasculitis*)
  - Nerves (*polyneuropathy* resulting from vasculitis, *compression* syndrome/CS 45, Fig. 122/)
  - Lungs (*fibrosis,* suspected *tumor* mass/Figs. 36a, 38, 39; CS 13/, pleuritis, *Caplan's* syndrome, which includes seropositive *RA* with progressive massive fibrosis or complicated *pneumoconiosis*)

In a male patient, 42 years, the pulmonary involvement with rheumatoid nodules and rheumatoid factor developed 1 year earlier than typical *RA* joint changes.

In a female patient, 54 years, *RF-* and *anti-CCP*-positive *RA, exudative pleuritis* developed with respiratory distress, resulting in emergency hospitalization and discharge with pleuritis of unknown etiology (what is unknown here?); the same occurred in a patient (CS 13) whereby the focal pulmonary changes (Figs. 36a, 39) had not been considered in the context of the underlying disease – seropositive *RA*.

- Heart (*myocarditis, exudative pericarditis* – dominant in one male patient with minimal arthritis)
- Kidneys (*glomerulonephritis, tubulopathies,* also medicinal; *secondary amyloidosis*)
- Liver (*adipose liver, hepatitis, drug toxicity* damage)
- Eyes (*keratoconjunctivitis sicca, iritis/iridocyclitis, uveitis* (Fig. 57)
- Blood and reticuloendothelial system (*anemia, splenomegaly, lymphadenopathy, neutropenia,* as in CS 68 in female patient with *Felty's* syndrome)
- Drug-induced toxicity of coxibs, NSAIDs, DMARDs, and TNF-blockers

The systemic aspects of rheumatic diseases (lead symptoms, syndromes, immunological activities) are to a large extent similar to *connective tissue diseases (CTD)* and *vasculitis/* Rheumatology Tree 2, *RCS,* Chap. 1.4/. Thereby, a solution should be found to the clinically relevant question whether *primary joint diseases* are involved, for example, *RA, chronic gouty arthritis* or *PsA* with systemic symptoms, which are most often attributable to *secondary vasculitis* or *metabolic* changes, or whether they are systemic rheumatic (*CTD, primary vasculitis*) or non-rheumatic (*tumors, autoimmune hepatitis, HIV,* etc.) diseases and conditions involving the joints.

A combination of *RA* and *SLE* with specific immunological markers is relatively rare, but possible. This difficulty is addressed in more detail in Sect. 2.

1.7
Deterioration in General Health

B symptoms (Chap. 8) often arise with inflammatory joint diseases (e.g., *RA*, acute *gout, infection*-related *arthritis*) on account of the following constellations:

- *Florid arthritis* and increased disease activity with polyarthritic involvement (almost with every episode)
- Highly aggressive disease (prompt onset and massive destruction)
- Serious restrictions to mobility (restricted active and passive movements) → Chap. 1.3
- Extra-articular system-organ involvement (Chap. 1.6).

1.8
Impaired Quality of Life

Such a syndrome, or such aspects, are ultimately the most important when it comes to joint diseases, since they involve highly detrimental effects on both *active* (inflammatory, which can therefore be influenced) and *passive* (cannot be influenced) mobility.

It is essential to question whether such impairments arise explicitly from the inflammatory aspects of the underlying disease or, as shown by CS 57, 59, 61, whether they are associated with a *secondary somatotropic pain* syndrome or *fibromyalgia*. The noninflammatory component of the restrictions to quality of life often plays the leading role and should thus be defined. The inflammatory factors, with a view to an impaired quality of life, should therefore be examined in closer detail.

Functional losses and inflammatory activity are closely correlated in *exudative/ inflammatory arthritis*. If *proliferative and fibrosing-ankylosing arthritis* predominate, the functional deficits – depending on the extent – can be influenced only to a limited degree by medication, or only by orthopedic approaches. With adequate therapy, the activity of the *arthritis* or functional deficits should, as a rule, abate and the quality of life improves accordingly. The scope and speed of such an improvement in *RA* and *PsA* is quantified during every study, but also routinely, by using the *HAQ (Health Assessment Questionnaire)*. The patients are thus asked standardized questions on their mobility, quality of life, and physical activity at home and on a daily basis, which are then quantified. Based on the responses, combined with other clinical and radiological data, the priority as regards the treatment of such diseases (currently MTX combined with biologicals) has been established and monitoring/differentiated therapy administered.

These factors were closely controlled with a view to the problems of insurance and pensions. Quality of life is therefore regarded as the primary objective and endpoint of the clinical, morphological, and pathophysiological changes and their socioeconomic consequences, as well as of all rheumatological and orthopedic treatment measures and studies.

Diseases of the Spine

2

2.1
Back Pain

This lead symptom is more significant and universal than *arthralgias*, and applies most predominantly to the problems of arthrological, as well as musculoskeletal and orthopedical disorders, described in this section. It is the initial diagnostic opening to further concepts, whereby consideration must always be given to neurological diseases and conditions, circulatory disorders, and virtually the entire scope of internal medicine (pulmonary, cardiological, gastrointestinal, nephrological, hematological, infectious diseases and conditions), but also psychosomatics (trauma) surgery and gynecology.

Once such diseases and conditions have been ruled out, the arthrological and vertebral syndromes, and above all the *back pain*, should be specifically addressed. The focus should be directed at the associated myelogenic (CS 46) and vascular syndromes reminiscent of *MS* (CS 18), which are seen in the neurological setting.

Back pain could be the initial signs of *vasculitis* (e.g., *Takayasu's arteritis*, cf. comments on Fig. 77 see in *RCS*, Chap. 2) or *tumor* disease. Arthrological back pain is not uncommon, for example, in spondyloarthropathy (*SpA*), under the guise of generalized *panalgesia* or *tendomyopathy* (*fibromyalgia*). The time taken on average to diagnose *SpA* is far too long and at the present time is a mean of 6.4 years. The characteristics of *arthrological back pain* are:

- Pain on movement or exertion
- Nocturnal pain with morning stiffness
- Restricted mobility, with and without pain
- Increased muscular tone (muscular tension)

Arthrological *back pain* affects all the anatomical structures of the spine, including the bones, soft tissue, and nerves (neuropathic components). Etiology: mostly degenerative (Chap. 2.3) and inflammatory (Chap. 2.2) diseases of the spine.

The features of back pain are linked to:

- The section of the backbone
- The many different etiologies

In their consideration, a distinction is made as given below.

E. Benenson, *Rheumatology*, Symptoms and Syndromes
DOI: 10.1007/978-1-84996-462-3_2, © Springer-Verlag London Limited 2011

2.1.1
Neck Pain

Cervicobrachialgias/CS 63/

- *Torticollis* ("stiff neck"), acute neck pain with asymmetrical positioning of the head and myogelosis, mostly with *uncovertebral arthrosis* (caused by a "draught")
- Subacute neck pain (DD *polymyalgia rheumatica* in patients over the age of 50)
- Chronic *cervical* syndrome (*pseudoradicular* pain syndrome), often with abnormal sensations (tingling and numbness) in one or more fingers and vegetative symptoms (dizziness, ocular disorders, tinnitus, etc.)
- Cervical radicular syndrome (*cervical nerve root compression* syndrome). Neurological deficits of sensitivity, motor function, and reflexes in the arms (C6–C7 most common; nerve roots C1–C4 hardly ever, except post-traumatic). In cervical spine block: typical "head inclination"
- Cervicomedullary syndrome (*cervical myelopathy*). Neurological deficits in the hands, arms, and legs (radicular syndrome with muscular atrophy, paresthesias, paraplegias)
- Headache ("*cervical migraine*"), episodic on exertion, also psychological, changes in the weather, *giant-cell arteritis*
- Dizziness (neurological investigation upon suspicion of *cervical arthritis* C1/C2)
- Pain in the shoulder/arm (DD *polymyalgia rheumatica*, *rotator cuff disease*, *impingement* syndrome, *Sudeck's* disease in the form of *shoulder-hand* syndrome in glenohumeral subluxation or after stroke)
- Pain with recumbency[1] or nocturnal pain (tumors, benign or malignant)
- Muscular tension[1] in the neck/shoulder region with radiation (*tendomyosis*)
- Pain with morning stiffness[1] (*AS*, Fig. 60: fresh syndesmophytes/left/are of absolute specificity to the disease)
- Localized bone pain[1] to the midline over osseous structures (fracture, bone necrosis, inflammatory, or neoplastic disorders)
- *RA* patients are a special risk group[24]: in roughly 17% arthritis of the atlanto-axial joints with or without pain (X-ray Fig. 60 and MRI diagnosis, CS 63), the following are involved:
  - Pannus formation (about 20%)
  - *Subluxations* (70%), atlanto-dental dislocation also with *PsA*
  - *Spondylodiscitis* below C2 (20%), as in Fig. 48a in thoracic spine region
  - *Myelocompression* (28%), as in Figs. 126 and 127a in the thoracic spine region

2.1.2
Thoracic Back Pain

Brachialgia/CS 17/

It is less often caused by rheumatic factors than the neck and low back pain, but has a broad spectrum of differential diagnostic patterns with regard to other non-rheumatological diseases and conditions.

---

[1]also applies to other sections of the spine

- *Rheumatic etiology*:

  - *AS* (the pain may occasionally intensify on breathing)/Fig. 117/
  - Tension in all the back muscles (*tendomyoses*)
  - *Spondylodiscitis* in AS (Fig. 48a) and other diseases
  - *Osteoporosis* with or without fractures (Figs. 125–127)
  - *Postural abnormalities*
  - *Scheuermann's* disease (adolescent kyphosis) most common *spinal* disease in adolescence

- *Non-rheumatological causes*:

  - Cardialgia (DD *angina pectoris, myocardial infarction*/CS 21/, *pericarditis*)
  - Pulmonary diseases (*pneumonia, pleuritis, pulmonary embolism*)
  - Infections (*Herpes zoster*), often during and after immunosuppression
  - Gastrointestinal diseases (*pancreatitis, ventricular* and *duodenal ulcer*)
  - Tumors (*plasmocytomas*, among others) and metastases
  - Psychogenic *rheumatism*

2.1.3
Low Back Pain

Lumbar syndrome (CS 69), radicular pain (sciatica)

Low back pain is the most common musculoskeletal complaint. Mechanical disorders are the most common causes of these syndromes:

- *Sciatica* (Acute low back pain or lumbago) – sudden onset of deep-seated pain in the lower back
- *Chronic back pain* (chronic lumbago) – radicular lumbar and/or nerve root compression syndrome → Chap. 3.12): lower back pain radiating into the gluteal muscles or iliac crest; depending on the area affected, localized tenderness, impaired sensitivity, and reflex deficits can be found (etiology: mostly prolapsed disc or lumbar spinal canal stenosis with distance-related pain, *Claudicatio spinalis*)
- *Cauda eguina* syndrome and/or *sacral root compression* syndrome (*radiating* pain, "saddle block anesthesia" as far as spinal transverse symptoms, impaired urination or defecation)
- *Aortitis* within the context of *Takayasu's arteritis* in *Aorta abdominalis* involvement (Figs. 77ab) or *AS*
- ❖ *Emergency surgery* with neurosurgical decompression (CS 46, Figs. 125–127)
  - *Pseudo-sciatica or pseudoradicular* syndrome (plus radiating pain, no neurological deficits)
  - *Ischialgia* pain, radiating as far as the legs or tips of the toes

When recording the patient's history, these two most common symptoms associated with back pain should be identified.

2.1.4
Noninflammatory Back Pain

(Mechanical disorders)

- Onset after the age of 40
- Occurrence connected with over-exertion (physical, psychosomatic), trauma, malpositioning
- As a rule, brief morning stiffness is described
- Deterioration following strain and over-exertion
- Inadequate improvement from nonsteroidal agents (NSAIDs)
- Particularly if there are neurological symptoms

Such features of *low back pain* could be attributed to functional conditions in the guise of noninflammatory *STR* (Chap. 3.4), or degenerative conditions and diseases (Chap. 2.3).

2.1.5
Inflammatory Back Pain

- Onset of back pain before the age of 40
- Persistent symptoms for over 3 months
- Pain in the early morning and when at rest (when waking early)
- Morning stiffness
- Improvement of pain and stiffness after moving and NSAIDs
- Lack of neurological symptoms

Such back pain is associated with SpA (Chap. 2.2)[8] and necessitates a strategic program of clinical and imaging examinations. To confirm the diagnosis, the intensity of the pain in the back and joints – measured by the patients on the VAS between 0 and 10 points – must be considered in combination with the intensity and duration of morning stiffness, as a parameter (*BASDAI: Bath Ankylosing Spondylitis Disease Activity Index)* of activity and severity in *AS*.

It must be remembered thereby that the specificity of the scores given by the patients using the *BASDAI* is relatively low (e.g., in patients with *fibromyalgia* or *panalgesia* (Chap. 3), and consequently a diagnosis is required which meets specific criteria. On that basis, these indices are used for monitoring therapy.

2.2
Spondyloarthropathy

This global term is used as a suspected diagnosis for *spinal* involvement, on account of the back pain and existing or identified concurrent diseases, and encompasses the inflammatory, degenerative, metabolic, and neurological diseases or conditions of the spine. Classification of *SpA*:

(a) Inflammatory *spondyloarthritis*
- Rheumatic *SpA*
  - Ankylosing spondylitis – *AS* (CS 15, 63; Figs. 60, 117, 124)
  - Inflammatory bowel disease (*Crohn's disease, Colitis ulcerosa*)
  - *Psoriasis, ReA*
  - Juvenile *SpA*
    - Differentiated form includes juvenile *SpA, ReA, PsA,* and arthritis with inflammatory bowel disease
    - Undifferentiated form includes *enthesitis-related arthritis, uveitis*
- *Spondylitis*, nonspecific and specific
  - *Spondylitis infectiosa (TB)*
- *Spondylodiscitis (AS,* CS 17) also with *CTD* (e.g., *MCTD*)
(b) Degenerative (*spondylarthrosis*)/Figs. 116, 118, 123/
(c) Metabolic
- *Osteoporosis* (CS 46)
- *Osteomalacia*
- Diabetic *spondylopathy* (Fig. 118)
- *Hypo-/hyperparathyroidism*
(d) Neurological
- *Tabes dorsalis*
- *Syringomyelia*

To formulate the diagnosis, this term is mostly used for metabolic and neurological problems, preferably just before confirming the diagnosis in line with specific criteria. In the case of inflammatory and degenerative changes, *spondyloarthritis* and *spondyloarthrosis* are used. All these (many others are not mentioned) diseases and conditions are essentially significant in clinical terms to rheumatology and orthopedics.

2.2.1
Spondyloarthritis

(Inflammatory *spine* diseases)

A group of diseases and conditions with lead symptoms:

- Inflammatory *back pain*
- Primary inflammatory diseases (*arthritis, enteropathies, TB, sepsis*)
- *Sacroiliitis* (Figs. 44–46, 124)
- *Spondylodiscitis* (Fig. 48a)
- Asymmetric joint involvement, primarily of the lower extremities (Fig. 24)
- Cutaneous (Figs. 84ab) and mucosal changes (potential association with above mentioned syndromes)

2.2.2
Spondylitis, Spondylodiscitis

Spondylitis is characterized by inflammation of the vertebrae, *spondylodiscitis* (Fig. 48a) by inflammation or tumorous destruction of the intervertebral discs and the adjacent base and top plates.

A differentiation is made between the following forms of *spondylitis*:

- Rheumatic (see above)
- Bacterial (abscess formation or osteomyelitis of a vertebral body), from
  - *Staphylococcus aurens*
  - *Streptococcus viridans*
  - Brucella
  - Tuberculosis bacteria
- Iatrogenic conditions, or conditions following
  - Nucleotomy
  - *Chemonucleolysis*
  - *Peridural anesthesia*
  - *Lumbar puncture*
- Tumorous (mostly resulting from metastasis)

Lead symptoms for bacterial and iatrogenic *spondylitis* or *spondylodiscitis*:

- Localized pain in the spinal column
- Primary localization: lower thoracic and upper lumbar spine
- Adaptive posture, stiffness
- Neurological deficits
- Serious signs of inflammation (*CRP, ESR* elevation)
- Historical evidence of previous or existing
  - Bacterial infections
  - TB
  - Sarcoidosis
  - HIV infection
  - Severe immunosuppression
  - Tumors
  - Therapeutic interventions

Diagnosis should be *confirmed* by means of the following procedures:

- X-ray
- Bone scan
- CT and MRI
- Vertebral body biopsy

2.2.3
Sacroiliitis

Sacroiliitis (Figs. 44–46, 124) is characterized by (a) symmetric destructive arthritis of the sacroiliac joints, with a distinction being made between

- Nonbacterial (rheumatic)
- Bacterial (*TB*) or septic (*Staphylococcus aurens*)

Clinically, there is a suspected diagnosis of *SpA* if the following are present:

- "Inflammatory pattern of back pain" in the lumbar region
- Tenderness in the sacroiliac joints
- Provoked pain (physical exertion, *Mennell's* test)
- Stiffness in the lumbar region
- Curvature in the lumbar spine (kyphosis, scoliosis)

Additionally, in bacterial *sacroiliitis*

- Predisposing factors (*HIV infection*, immunosuppression, *TB, sepsis*)
- Serious signs of inflammation (CRP, ESR elevation)
- Acute (after 2–3 weeks) and widespread destruction

Confirmation of diagnosis by

- X-ray (Figs. 44, 60, 117, 124)
  - A "colorful picture" of
    - Widening or narrowing of joint space (Figs. 44, 124)
    - Sclerosis (Figs. 117, 124)
    - Erosions or *osteolysis* (Fig. 45)
    - *Ankylosis*, partial or full (cf. staging, Fig. 124)
  - Symmetric changes (mostly *AS*, Figs. 117, 119, 124)
  - Asymmetric (also with other forms of *SpA*, Fig. 46)
- Bone scintigraphy (in particular, relatively specific asymmetric enhancement in sacroiliac joint)
- CT (Figs. 45, 118, 126, 127ab) and MRI (Figs. 46, 121)
- Vertebral body biopsy

2.3
Degenerative Spinal Diseases or Mechanical Disorders of the Spine

Such diseases are most common in humans and are mostly treated by orthopedic specialists. They involve changes in the intervertebral discs, vertebrae, and often uncovertebral, sacroiliac joints and paraspinous ligaments. The classic signs of disc and joint degeneration (osteophyte formation in the joints, fissuring, and curvatures) can best be verified by radiological, CT, and MRI scans. They involve, primarily the following.

2.3.1
Disc and Paraspinous Ligament Disorders

- *Chondrosis (Chondrosis intervertebralis)* – diminishment of the intervertebral space as a result of sintering of the disc or loss of height in the disc space (Figs. 123, 127a)
- *Osteochondrosis (Osteochondrosis intervertebralis)* – chondrosis + irregularities and condensation, that is, sclerotic reaction of the adjacent vertebral bodies and/or facing top and base plates, with formation of spondylophytes (Fig. 116)
- Diffuse idiopathic skeletal hyperostosis/*DISH/(Forestier's* disease) refers to calcification and ossification of paraspinous ligaments – a special form influenced by metabolism: serious ventral hyperostoses (*NB*: *no syndesmophytes*) found radiologically, almost always in the lower thoracic spine with stiffening of this area (Fig. 118)
- *Intervertebral disc herniation* causes nerve impingement and inflammation that result in radicular pain (sciatica), often with neurologic deficits
- *Osteochondrosis juvenilis (Scheuermann's* disease)

2.3.2
Spondyloarthrosis

- *Spondylosis (Spondylosis deformans)* – formation of marginal spikes (spondylophytes) on the vertebral bodies (Figs. 116, 123, 127b)
- *Spondylarthrosis (Spondylarthrosis deformans)* – diminishment of the small vertebral joints with increased sclerosis and formation of marginal spikes (the same characteristics as for the joints in the extremities)
- *Baastrup's* disease (constitutional enhancement of the spinous processes, intensified lordosis)
- *Spondylolisthesis* is the anterior displacement of a vertebral body in relation to the underlying vertebra and usually secondary to *osteochondrosis*
- *Uncovertebral arthrosis* (disorders of the neck) – restriction of *Foramina intervertebralia* with potential *nerve root* syndrome and impairment of *Arteria* and *Plexus vertebralis*
- *Spinal canal stenosis* (Fig. 126) caused in certain circumstances by *Claudicatio spinalis* (Chap. 9.2.5): pain on exertion and neurological symptoms in the legs, possibly dramatic ("numbness in the legs"), but transient

Such radiomorphological signs are not necessarily consistent with local symptoms and more likely serve as an exclusion diagnosis for nondegenerative spinal disease (bacterial, rheumatic, traumatic, malformations, tumors, metastases).

2.4
Involvement of the Joints in Diseases of the Spine

Involvement of the joints in diseases of the spine (as well as a history of such) is deduced from the manifestation of the back pain. Conversely, such joint problems indicate the type of *spinal* involvement and can even occur prior to the back pain itself.

2.4.1
Arthritis

(Inflammatory pattern in *spinal* diseases)

- *Mono-/oligoarthritis*, possibly erosive with destruction and ankylosis/Figs. 21, 24, 119/within a short period; occurring as the initial symptom of *SpA* in 20–40% of cases (CS 8). In one of our patients, a 16-year-old male, full ankyloses developed in both hips during the first 6 months of *AS*:
    - Predominantly in the large joints near the trunk/hips, knees, and shoulders/(rhisomelic form)
    - Asymmetric, rarely symmetric *hip arthritis* (Fig. 119)
    - Mostly not destructive
- Following *concomitant syndromes*:
    - Ocular involvement (*Epi-/Scleritis*, Fig. 57), could precede *AS*
    - Urogenital problems of an inflammatory nature
    - Heel pain (*calcaneopathy*) and other forms of *enthesitis* (Figs. 98, 108, 120)
    - Neurological deficits (due to *atlanto-dental arthritis* and dislocations in *SpA*) or *myelocompression* with paraplegia, as in Figs. 126, 127a, CS 46

2.4.2
Osteoarthritis

(Noninflammatory pattern in spinal diseases)

- *Generalized OA* of the large and small joints (Chap. 1.4)
- No concurrent inflammatory symptoms or history thereof

2.4.3
MRI-Confirmed Syndromes

- *Osteitis* (Fig. 102), *synchondritis* (symphysis, Figs. 119, 120) or sternum, *perichondritis manubrii sternalis*, cf. comments on CS 21 in **RCS**, Chap. 2
- Aseptic necrosis (Fig. 121)

- Secondary *arthritis* and *periarthritis* (Fig. 106)
- *Atlanto-dental arthritis* (this area is presented in Fig. 60 and the relevant clinical findings in CS 63) and dislocations

2.5
Malpositioning and Curvature of the Spine

An abnormal profile to the *spine* has various components which can possibly be combined:

- Constitutional or idiopathic
- Age-related (*osteoporosis*)
- Disease-related (*SpA, spondylosis, spondylolisthesis*)

The *acquired malpositioning* of the spine is expressed by a diminishment in height, axial deviations, blockades, or pelvic asymmetry, and are associated with:

- *Osteoporosis* (primary and cortisone-induced) due to shrinking of the spine (Figs. 125, 127a)
- *AS* (Figs. 117, 124) and *osteochondrosis* (Figs. 116, 118, 123)
- *Spondylodiscitis* (sterile, septic, tumorous) due to diminishment of the intervertebral space (Fig. 48a)
- *Kyphosis* of neck and thorax sections (in *SpA*, most commonly *AS* and *spondyloses*), also in what is known as *Scheuermann's* kyphosis (impaired growth in the top and base plates with cuneiform, deformed vertebral bodies)
- Spondylolistesis reveals *lordosis* with a "step off"
- Pelvic malpositioning arises from differences in leg length and contractures of the hip joints (*OA* of the *hip*, Fig. 97; *aseptic osteonecrosis*, Fig. 121)

Curvatures of the *spine* and static disorders (support reaction!) are characterized inevitably by *back pain*, which, above all, is almost always attributable to concomitant *osteochondrosis, tendomyoses* with facet joint blocks (*pseudoradicular* syndrome), and *compression* syndrome.

The *most common curvatures* and profile disorders of the spine are:

- *Kyphosis* (round/flat back)
- *Lordosis*
- *Scoliosis*, structural and functional, due to
- Differences in the *lengths of the extremities*

At the same time as vertebral symptoms, pulmonary (restrictive ventilatory disorders, *pulmonary hypertension* in scoliosis) or myelogenic (spinal overextension with severe kyphosis) factors must be considered.

2.6
Extra-articular Manifestations and Associated Diseases

Such factors play a decisive role in the diagnosis, therapy, and prognosis of *spinal* diseases (Chap. 2.4).

2.6.1
Extra-articular Manifestations

(See Chaps. 1.6 and 10)

- Ocular (*iritis-/iridocyclitis, uveitis, epi-/scleritis*, Fig. 57)
- Cardiovascular (*aortitis, aortic insufficiency*, arrhythmias)
- Pulmonary (diminished vital capacity, restrictive ventilatory disorders, *pulmonary fibrosis, Caplan's* syndrome/association of the seropositive *RA* and *pneumoconiosis/*)
- Renal (interstitial *nephritis, amyloidosis*)
- Intestinal (*Crohn's* disease, Colitis ulcerosa, infections)
- Neurological (*compression* syndrome/CS 46/, atlas dislocation, *cauda equina* syndrome)
- Drug-induced toxicity of coxibs, NSAIDs, DMARDs, and TNF-blockers

2.6.2
Associated Diseases and Conditions

- Curvatures, hereditary and acquired (kyphosis, lordosis, scoliosis)
- *Psoriasis vulgaris* and *pustulosa* (Figs. 84, 110–111, 129b)
- Urogenital diseases (*urethritis, balanitis*)
- Inflammatory bowel diseases (*Crohn's* disease, Colitis ulcerosa)
- Degenerative or inflammatory joint changes and such whose nature is likewise a key to diagnosis of the respective changes in the spine

2.7
Deterioration in General Health

The related symptoms are seen to be highly relevant in *joint* and *spinal* diseases, and are remarkable primarily in inflammatory diseases due to:

- Fever and more severe signs of inflammation (with florid polyarthritic involvement of *RA, Still's* disease, *SpA, inflammatory arthropathies, septic arthritis*)
- Considerable restrictions to mobility, particularly active painful movements (*gout arthritis, aseptic necrosis, Sudeck's* syndrome) or in marked *spinal kyphosis*, several

contractures and *ankylosis* of the musculoskeletal system (impairment to passive movements) or due to *compression* syndrome (Chap. 3.12)
- Systemic extra-articular symptoms (Chaps. 1.6 and 10)
- Serious concomitant diseases (*Crohn's* disease, *Colitis ulcerosa*, infections, *sepsis*)

If there is no clinical correlate to the deterioration in *general health*, and the history is short, a broad therapeutic investigation in the context of systematic screening for *tumors, metastases,* and *infections* should be instigated (Chap. 13.3).

2.8 Restrictions to Quality of Life

This important syndrome, involving diseases of the joints and spine, has a significant influence on the burden suffered by affected patients. In some diseases the full burden of the disease is difficult to gauge on account of the often inconsistent correlation between (radio) morphology and symptoms, for example, in *osteoporosis* (*spine* sintering or fracturing) or in destructive forms of *arthritis* (Chap. 1.3.4). The quality of life is measured on a scale of functional loss and is closely monitored, in fact as part of study routine (using specific questionnaires, for example, *BASMI: Bath Ankylosing Spondylitis Metrology Index*) or on account of difficulties concerning insurance and pensions.

Quality of life is regarded as an endpoint of clinical, morphological, and pathophysiological changes and their socioeconomic consequences, as well as a *primary objective* of all rheumatological and orthopedic treatment measures and studies.

Soft-Tissue Rheumatism and Related Disorders

Soft-Tissue Rheumatism (*STR*) is a global term encompassing different diseases and conditions which play varied roles in all soft-tissue structures. This group of disorders (synonyms: *extra-articular rheumatism, soft-tissue disorders or diseases*) plus damage from overexertion is certainly one of the most common problems experienced and handled in medical routine. Such problems are inadequately addressed by medical training, if at all. The triggers for *STR* are global and multifarious.

The most common are:[15, 22]

- Overuse and misload (e.g., on account of spinal disease)
  - Trauma, often sport-related
  - Neural
  - Psychogenic
  - Influence of cold, damp, and changes in the weather
- Hormonal
- Metabolic factors

However, this more outpatient-oriented aspect tends to limit – considerably in fact – quality of life and capacity to work, but prognostically has a more favorable outlook than inflammatory rheumatic diseases.

This group of disorders involves a number of clinically and pathogenetically varied diseases and conditions, mostly with no underlying inflammatory involvement (*primary STR*) or presenting as concomitant symptoms to inflammatory rheumatic diseases (*secondary STR*). Furthermore, such multifarious, inhomogeneous entities should be attributed not only to the soft-tissue structures of the connective tissue, but also to the most commonly affected anatomical pain regions.

The most common entities of this group should be regarded more as conditions and less often as diseases (Rheumatology Tree 1, see *RCS*, Chap. 1.3), and can be divided into an inflammatory and a noninflammatory form as

- Associated with the relevant joint (*arthritis* and *osteoarthritis* [*OA*]) and spinal diseases (*SpA* and *spondylosis*)
- Induced by local mechanical factors or by overuse

- Caused by nerve damage
- Systemic diseases

In *STR*, all extra-articular layers can basically be affected and, accordingly, be differentiated only by MRI upon suspicion of changes in the deep-seated structures.

Common lead clinical syndromes and symptoms:

- Pain, regional or diffuse
- Tenderness, localized
- Stiffness and restricted mobility, mostly local
- Muscle strain, local or systemic

In the case of *arthritis* and *SpA*, active screening for concomitant symptoms in the periarticular and other structures of the musculoskeletal system should be instigated. The most important syndromes, as shown, are initially considered in association with anatomical connective tissue structures and then with the nature of pathophysiological changes. Such reasoning is important to the diagnosis and therapy of the many polydimensional changes in *STR*. In healthcare regulations, which are used as guidelines for physical therapy, the above mentioned lead syndromes or symptoms of *STR*, the diseased structures of the connective tissue, and therapy are consolidated.

3.1
Cutaneous/Subcutaneous Tissue (Nodules)

Nodules often develop and are of great diagnostic significance. The nodules develop in a number of diseases, as diverse inflammatory reactions in the subcutaneous tissue (*panniculitis*) or deposits (*tophi*, calcinates), or primarily in the bones (*Heberden's* and *Bouchard's* nodes) or tendon sheaths (*ganglia*), or in *vasculitis* (Chap. 9.4.2, Fig. 33).

3.1.1
"Rheumatoid Nodules"

"Rheumatoid nodules" (Figs. 3, 35, 80, 104, 122ab, 129c) are extra-articular symptoms of *seropositive RA* (found very seldom in seronegative *RA*), appearing as round or oval, hard, and mostly painless nodes of varying sizes (0.5–3 cm). They mostly appear as subcutaneous and periostal, tumor-like structures (Fig. 122ab) on the extensor sides of the elbows, fingers, and feet (Figs. 3, 80, 104), Achilles' tendon, seldom visceral, in the internal organs such as the lungs (Figs. 36a, 38), pleura with effusions, and eyes.

Such nodules should be regarded as an indicator of *vasculitis* with central fibrinoid necrosis, characteristic in 10–30% of seropositive *RA* patients (a main diagnostic criterion), posing serious diagnostic difficulties (CS 13, 45). As a rule, they are associated with a highly active disease – ultimately even with systemic (e.g., *polyneuropathy*) or local (*compression* syndrome [CS 45], *ulceration* [Fig. 55], tendon rupture, infection) symptoms – but could not only be reduced, but also appear under MTX therapy. B-cell targeted therapy with rituximab could considerably reduce the rheumatoid nodules. DD "Churg-Strauss granuloma" in RF-positive *WG* and *CSS* (CS 72, Chap. 11.2).

3.1.2
Tophi

Tophi are urate deposits (sodium urate crystals) with persistently high uric acid levels in the tissues (joints, cartilage, tendons) and signify a chronic phase of *gout arthritis* (Fig. 13, 114). Such deposits appear most often in bones near to the joints in the region of the toes (CS 55, Fig. 130b), the synovial membrane, but also the bursae (*bursitis* in *gout*) and the helix of the ear ("gout pearls"). White or whitish-yellow, subcutaneous tophi can vary in size and be perforated. If the bone is affected (Fig. 130b), *destructive arthritis* develops almost without any pain and with very minimal activity or no local activity whatsoever. On the other hand, if *tophi* are deposited in the tendon sheaths or tendon attachments, they cause painful movement deficits necessitating surgery. Invariably, this will involve certain complications (Fig. 115, CS 43).

The tophi and *gout arthritis* in general almost always pose a diagnostic problem, both in the very young (CS 55, in a 10-year-old girl, despite the typically "male" course [18], on account of being extremely rare) and in the elderly, since it is not often easy to differentiate between *OA* with *synovitis* and *RA* (Fig. 13; CS 47, Fig. 130ab) when the uric acid concentration is often elevated. Without *tophi* the diagnosis of acute gout arthritis should be made because of the typical patterns in the gout infestation (Fig. 13). *Tophi* could largely be reversed by applying optimal, long-term gout therapy (diet, allopurinol, benzbromarone, and particularly febuxostat, a *novel non-purine selective inhibitor of xanthine oxidase*).

3.1.3
Heberden's and Bouchard's Nodes

Heberden's (DIP joints, Figs. 3, 4, 8, 81, 89) and Bouchard's nodes
(PIP joints, Figs. 4, 81, 128ab) are highly specific signs of *OA* (Chap. 1.4) and should be isolated in the activated state from rheumatoid nodules or tophi. This can be achieved by radiological examinations (compare Figs. 8, 128b against Fig. 9a). Certain difficulties arise if both cases are found in the form of destructive changes, particularly with PIP involvement (Figs. 4, 81, 128a, CS 28).

The differentiation of DIP and PIP *inflammatory OA* from *arthritis* of the fingers, above all in *RA* and *PsA*, appears to be the most difficult problem in terms of arthrology, also to specialist colleagues. This is the case, for example, in the female patient with MCP arthritis (Figs. 128ab) and low-titer RF who was referred with suspected *RA*; the same applies to Fig. 81, CS 28, whereby the patient was treated in fact with MTX.

Here it is essential to capture the entire *pattern of involvement*, and above all the condition in the MCP joints and wrists, which are affected specifically by *RA* and other inflammatory joint diseases (Figs. 5, 9ab, 21, 28, 35, 40, 49ab, 58–59, 64, 80, 104, 129ac) and thereby signify the distinction from *OA*. Individual patients can of course have two diseases, as can be deduced from Figs. 3, 9b, 42, 89.

3.1.4
Calcification

Calcification (Fig. 18) is a syndrome in different diseases and also has a certain nosological specificity, irrespective of localization, namely in the the following:

- Elbows, fingers, and *prepatellar bursa*, such calcification occur with calcinosis (*Calcinosis interstitialis*) within the context of *SSc* (*Thibierge–Weissenbach* syndrome) or more frequently in *C (alcinosis) REST* syndrome (Chap. 9.4.3). This virtually disease-specific calcinosis could cause, in certain circumstances, local inflammation or ulceration.
- Tendons (*Tendinosis calcarea* or *calcific tendititis*), e.g., Achilles' tendon, plantar aponeurosis (*calcaneal spur*, Fig. 108), *M. flexor hallucis brevis*
- Muscles (*myositis ossificans*), diagnosable on account of palpable hardening or calcification and by imaging methods (conventional X-rays, CT and bone scans) – this also applies to other localizations. Traumatic, neurological disorders, and *PM/DM* can be given as the cause.
- Shoulders (*calcific tendinitis*), developing as a result of chronic inflammation, trauma, torn fascia, and tendon sheaths
- Kidneys (*nephrocalcinosis*), more often in *Sjögren's* syndrome or *SLE* (Fig. 105)
- Vessels are subject to calcification due to chronic inflammation (*vasculitis*) and *thrombophilia* in *Takayasu's arteritis, antiphospholipid* syndrome, *SLE*.

3.1.5
Ganglions

Ganglions (*Menisceal cysts*) are characterized by elastic, tumorous nodes in the connective tissue much like *bursitis* (Figs. 28, 42), namely in the region of the joints, fasciae, tendon sheaths (Fig. 104), and menisci. They are most commonly seen in the wrists (next to extensor tendon of thumb) and knee joints and cause strictly localized (pressure) pain and restricted movements, possibly inducing a *compression* syndrome (*ulnar nerve*).

Rare forms of nodule formation are the *dermatofibromas* (benign skin tumors of spindle cells on the arm and legs, e.g., in *SLE*, and other diseases of immune dysregulation), *fibroma* (elastic subcutaneous nodes in the fingers), and *osteoma* or *sarcoma* of the fascia (suspected diagnosis prior to surgery in a female patient with *RA*, CS 45, Figs. 112ab, which could not be confirmed).

3.2
Subcutaneous Tissue

3.2.1
Panniculitis

Such conditions are characterized initially by exudative and later fibrosing or granulomatous inflammation within the subcutaneous fatty tissue, manifesting them as

- *Primary* (seldom) in the form of lipogranulomatosis or *Pfeifer–Weber–Christian* disease, a systemic disease with fat necroses in the subcutaneous tissue and rarely the internal organs. The *lead symptoms* are:
  - Diffuse subcutaneous changes (painful inflammatory nodes with scarring)
  - B symptoms (Chaps. 2.7 and 8)
  - Organ involvement (pancreas and possibly other organs)
- *Secondary* (common)
  - Infections, often *yersiniosis* (Fig. 6, CS 1; Fig. 109, CS 40)
  - *CTD* and *vasculitis* (Chap. 9.4.1, Figs. 27, 71) – *erythrodermic panniculitis* or *Lupus profundus* as an erythema of brick-red complexion with no keratosis
  - Drug-induced (Fig. 16)
  - *Paraneoplasia* (in one of our patients with chronic leukemia, morphologically confirmed symmetrical panniculitis, as in Fig. 27, on the feet and lower legs)
  - T- and B-cell *lymphoma*
  - *Sarcoidosis* (Fig. 83)
  - *Subcutaneous phlegmona* (in a patient with *RA*, initially believed to be *erythema nodosum*)
  - Pancreatic diseases
  - *Alpha-1 antitripsin deficiency*

Most common clinical variant:

- *Erythema nodosum* (Fig. 109) is the most common form of *panniculitis*, regarded as *vasculitis* (histologically there was a perivascular reaction).

Clinically:

- Often painful, red, hard, and sometimes only palpable nodes (diameter ranging from 0.5 cm to 10 cm) and/or plaques in the subcutaneous fatty tissue, mostly in the lower extremities
- Unilateral or bilateral above the shin, on the extensor sides of the lower extremities and ankles
- Such changes are mostly recurrent (CS 40), self-limiting with regression and no scarring, within 4–6 weeks

The *causes* can be divided into two groups, should be considered in sequence, and be ruled out:

- Infections
  - Streptococcal pharyngitis
  - Yersinia (Fig. 6) and other intestinal infections, *borreliosis*
- Systemic diseases:
  - *Sarcoidosis* (Fig. 90; Fig. 83 shows no erythema in this histologically confirmed disease)
  - *CTD* (*SLE*, Fig. 27; *MCTD*, Fig. 71)
  - Systemic *vasculitis* (*microscopic polyangiitis*, Fig. 12)
  - Chronic bowel diseases (*Crohn's* disease, *Colitis ulcerosa*)
  - Pancreatitis

- *Paraneoplasias* (pancreatic carcinoma)
- Systemic panniculitis (*Pfeifer–Weber–Christian* disease)
- Drug toxicity (antibiotics, contraceptives)

3.2.2
Panniculosis/Cellulitis

This is not one of the inflammatory forms of subcutaneous change and is characterized by widespread thickening of the subcutaneous tissue, with the appearance of large pores ("orange peel" skin), whereby the skin is difficult to manipulate, pinch sensitive, and often feels warm to the touch.

Lead symptoms: It is mostly women who are affected, and often underlying psychosomatic factors should be evaluated. *Fibromyalgia*-type concomitant symptoms appear, accordingly (Chap. 3.5).

Most commonly, such changes occur in the following areas:

- Shoulder and neck
- Flanks and hips
- Outer side of upper arms and upper legs
- Inner side of knee joints

3.2.3
Dercum's Disease

Dercum's disease (*Adipositas dolorosa neurolipomatosis*) is a special nodular form of *panniculosis*, taking the form of small subcutaneous nodules measuring up to 5 cm in diameter which are diffuse and painful, with fat necroses. In one of our female patients with *fibromyalgia* syndrome, these nodules were examined histologically: "numerous necrobiotically modified adipocytes can be seen in the upper corium. The collagenous fibers also reveal necrobiotic changes. There are numerous lymphocytes and macrophages. Diagnosis: the finding is highly consistent with *Dercum's* disease."

Rheumatological investigation ensues on two grounds, initially to explain the existing, diffuse, long-term symptoms of pain and fatigue, which can only be distinguished from *fibromyalgia* due to the existence of such nodules, and secondly, to decide on the necessity of biopsy of the nodules (not essential, unless other conditions are a possibility).

3.3
Tendons and Tendon Sheaths

3.3.1
Tendinopathy and Tendinitis

Such is the description for the diseases in these structures – a global term for inflammatory, seldom necrotic changes in the tendons (*tendinitis, tendovaginitis*) and paratenon (*peritendinitis*) as well as mechanically and metabolically induced tendon degeneration (*tendinosis, tendomyosis*), whereas clinically and morphologically (by MRI) it is difficult to distinguish between such changes[4] (Figs. 63, 95, 102, 106).

Clinical signs of *tendinopathy* or *tendinitis* and *peritendinitis*:

- Pain is mostly very localized, to some extent severe
- Pain in a certain area of the joint cleft and externally along the length of the tendon
- Run-in pain (on first movement, with alleviation of the pain thereafter)
- Pain from one movement, often only at one level against resistance (when tensing the muscles), e.g., the arm is actively abducted into an overhead position (*rotator cuff tendinitis* is the major cause of a painful shoulder)
- Pain from pressure and pulling along the length of the affected tendon
- Adaptive posture in the joints to relieve the tendon
- Pain-free variant (e.g., in *tendinitis* of the flexor tendons of the fingers, Fig. 63)
- Signs of inflammation (reddening, swelling, warmth) in florid *tendinitis* (as a rule in *ReA*, *gout*, bacterial *infection*, constant occupation, or play with computer mouse)
- Lack of symptoms of impingement syndrome (e.g., *carpal tunnel* syndrome)
- The most common localizations of *tendinitis*:
  - Shoulder (Chaps. 3.13, 6.1, Fig. 106)
  - Hand (long flexor tendon, Figs. 63, 95)
  - Hips (*M. piriformis*)
  - Dorsum of the foot and heel (Achilles' tendon, *M. posterior longus*)

3.3.2
Tenosynovitis

Tenosynovitis (Fig. 104 right) is the inflammatory form of *tendinopathy* within the tenosynovium or peritenon (peritendinitis), either with effusion (exudative-proliferative forms) or without (dry form), and appears with

- *Tendinitis* symptoms mentioned above, plus
  - Crepitation, rubbing, and creaking of the affected tendon
  - Swelling and/or palpable effusions along the tendon
  - "Trigger or *snapping finger*," or snapping phenomenon (*tendopathy nodosa*)
  - Tendon of the thumb (*tendovaginitis stenosans de Quervain*)
  - Calcification in the periarticular structures (*tendinosis calcarea*)
  - The (sub) acute functional deficits of the fingers (Fig. 63) can be regarded as spontaneous ruptures of the extensor and flexor tendons of the wrists and finger joints, which in turn could be the outcome of chronic *tenosynovitis* in *RA* and *OA* as well as the local application of corticosteroid crystal suspension.

In the clinical consideration of such problems, the causal and/or pathophysiological factors are of great importance, i.e., how they developed: on the one hand, through *primary* mechanical influences (unilateral activity, certain types of sport, work inappropriate to one's own resilience, psychological and physical influences), or even *secondary* factors within the context of existing inflammatory-rheumatic, endocrinological, and metabolic disease. In the case of both these causes, the inflammatory component could play the pivotal role while the mechanically induced changes are to be evaluated more as noninflammatory. The development of such symptoms in *RA* and other systemic forms of *arthritis* are described as *tenosynovialitis*. These, in turn, influence the changes in other structures, e.g., *carpal tunnel* syndrome (Chap. 3.12.1) with *tenosynovitis* of the long flexor tendons of the hand or *impingement* syndrome (Chap. 4.1).

In morphological diagnosis, with the sometimes complicated concomitant symptoms, the deciding factor is firstly arthrosonography and then – for greater specificity and sensitivity (almost 100%) – MRI (Figs. 102, 106).

3.4
Muscles/Fasciae: Localized Tendomyopathies and Tendomyoses

These are the most common causes of "rheumatic" pain and *local myofascial pain* syndrome. Noninflammatory, highly localized (according to muscular localization) muscular changes are predominant, in the form of strain (the subjective sensation popularly known as "seized muscles") and muscular hypertension (a decisive pathogenetic factor).

Lead symptoms:

- Local, possibly severe pain around the back and the extremities
- *Trigger points* entail "myofascial," transmitted pain in the respective muscular regions which is not always highly demarcated, often with palpable muscular hardening, paresthesias, *myasthenia*, and/or vegetative concomitant symptoms (not to be confused with *tender points* in *fibromyalgia* → Chap. 3.5)
- Most commonly affected are the *M. trapezius, M. pectoralis*, paralumbar musculature (in *pseudoradicular* syndrome → Chap. 3.12.1), and thigh/upper arm (in *OA* with *synovitis* and *shoulder pain* → Chaps. 1.4.2, 4.1)
- Orofascial pain is a dull, constant with local tenderness in the muscles of the jaws and difficulty in opening the mouth
- Acute and chronic, recurrent forms (with persistence of the triggers, e.g., poor posture, overload, psychic factors)
- Intensification of pain from static effort, cold, damp, fatigue, and psychological factors or stress
- Improvement from heat, movement, and physiotherapy
- Normal laboratory values
- Prognostically, self-limiting and benign on the whole

Most common localizations:

- Supraspinatus tendon
- Infraspinatus tendon
- Multilocal occurrence of calcereous deposits

3.5
Muscles/Attachments (Generalized Tendomypathy or Fibromyalgia)

This is one of the most common and insidious diseases, also known as *diffuse pain syndrome* or *myofascial* or *somatogenic pain* syndrome, *chronic fatigue* syndrome, or *muscular rheumatism*. It is mostly women aged 25–55 years who are affected.

What is remarkable with this (sub) acute disease is an enormous, as yet unexplained discrepancy between the massive degree of suffering and the objectifiable symptoms. It should initially be regarded as a condition (*secondary fibromyalgia*) in other, partly rheumatic diseases (inflammatory/CS 57, 61/, degenerative and tumorous/CS 59/), and only once other diseases have been ruled out over the course should it – depending on the lead symptoms – be described as *primary fibromyalgia* or *fatigue* syndrome, or clearly definable *panalgesia* syndrome. The nature of the condition is chronically refractive and, in fact, tends to improve after the age of 60.

Lead symptoms:

- *"Pain everywhere,"* diffuse (more than 3 months) in the back and extremities, to some extent with movement deficits and as intense as a supposed episode of inflammatory rheumatic disease (CS 57)
- Typical, thereby, is a prolonged inability to work (CS 57) which is not commensurate with the minimal activity of the underlying disease (*PsA*), or many years of a continued need for strong painkillers in a patient with *RA* (CS 61), or an undetectable morphological correlate for the pain in the hands of a young computer scientist
- Local multiple pressure points in typical locations (*tender points*)
- *Fatigue* syndrome (resulting in a 32-year-old female patient being wheelchair-bound), associated with Epstein–Barr virus infection or antibodies
- Colorful, mixed pattern of symptoms, the majority of which are general, vegetative, and psychosomatic disorders which can hardly be differentiated from the severe underlying disease (CS 59)
- These patients have a disproportionately high rate of doctor's appointments and often undergo unnecessary surgical interventions (laparotomy is 4 times more common than in the normal population)
- No inflammatory signs, nonarticular and no increase in *CK*
- *Neither morphological nor neurological correlate*, but psychosomatic disorders in such patients with a serious drop in performance
- Continuous need for painkillers with minimal disease activity (CS 61) is mostly suggestive of *diffuse somatogenic pain* syndrome
- Nonetheless, mainly organic as well as muscular diseases and conditions should be ruled out prior to making a diagnosis (Chap. 9.6).

Virtually identical symptoms with diffuse tenderness, i.e., beyond the *tender points*, primarily suggest *panalgesia* or *chronic pain* syndrome or *somatoform pain-processing* disorders. Such patients require a multimodal treatment concept, as is available at pain clinics.

3.6
Insertion Site

3.6.1
Enthesiopathy, Insertion Tendopathy, or Enthesitis

Here we have inflammatory, hyperostotic, and resorptive changes in the multilayered anatomical structures (a connective tissue complex of tendons, tendon sheaths, bursae, per-
ichondrium, and periost), the enthesitis is the site of tendinous or ligamentous attachment
to the bone. There are two main causes for *enthesiopathy*: one involves chronic, local,
mechanical, and often physical overexertion, and the other, inflammatory systemic spinal
and joint diseases (Fig. 102, CS 37).

The term *enthesitis* is characterized in association with *SpA* by erosive, inflammatory
lesions that may eventually undergo ossification and has the *following pattern*:

- Several localizations, particularly in areas which are not under a great deal of mechani-
cal strain, e.g., sternum-costal cartilage transition (Chap. 4.2)
- Could in fact occur prior to the *back pain*, alone or combined with *mono-/
oligoarthritis*
- Correlated to disease activity
- In such a case the term is *"enthesitis-related arthritis"* – a form of undifferentiated
SpA, most commonly with *PsA* or *"juvenile SpA"* (Figs. 21–23, CS 8), enthesitis can
help differentiate *PsA* from *RA*
- Localized predominantly and almost specifically to predilection sites:
  - Spinous processes (cervical C1/C2, C7/T1 and lumbal T12/L1, L5/S1 spine)
  - Parasternal, *Manubrium sterni* (*synchondrosis*, Fig. 69)
  - *Symphysis pubis* (*symphysitis*, Figs. 119, 120)
  - *Trochanter major*
  - Knee (Fig. 25)
  - Achilles' tendon (Fig. 102)
  - Plantar ligaments (*plantar fasciitis*, Fig. 98)

An *enthesiopathy* index has proven successful for follow-up monitoring and therapeutic
studies.

Clinical:

- Pain in the tendon attachments when tensing the respective muscle
- Increased muscle tone and/or contractures
- Severe pain at rest in the acute stage, with adaptive posture
- Exclusion of *pseudo-/radicular* syndromes and *sacroiliitis*
- Tenderness at the predilection sites (see above), namely in the following forms:
  - *Epicondylitis humeri radialis* (*tennis elbow*) and *ulnaris* (*Golfer's elbow*)
  - *Trochanter major* (*trochanteritis, trochanteric bursitis*)
  - Patellar tendon (*bursitis prepatellaris*, Fig. 25)

- Achilles' tendon (synonym: posterior *calcaneal spur*, Fig. 108)
- Plantar (*plantar fasciitis* → Chap. 3.7; Fig. 98, CS 36)
- Supraspinatus tendon (*shoulder blade margin* syndrome, Fig. 106)
- *Os pubis* "*Grazilis* syndrome," Fig. 120)

3.6.2
Fibroostitis or Fibroostosis

Fibroostitis or fibroostosis (inflammatory and noninflammatory *calcaneal spur*) is a radiological diagnosis (Fig. 108) of *enthesiopathy* (Chap. 3.7.2) associated in the case of pain in the heel with *plantar fasciitis* (Fig. 98, same female patient); there was no pain after successfully treating the *fibroostitis* (Fig. 99).

3.7
Fasciae

Here, above all, we see *fasciitis* syndrome (Chap. 9.4.4) and isolated fascial involvement (local or diffuse forms), or also muscle involvement (*myofascial pain* syndrome), which can be regarded in the context of *tendomyosis* or *generalized tendomyopathy*, or even *paraneoplasia* (Chap. 5).

Lead symptoms of *fasciitis*:

- Diffuse pain and localized tenderness (depending on the extent)
- Acute pain (in the case of ruptures)
- Reddening and swelling
- Softer tumor (muscular hernias in the upper arm, lower leg with fascial lacunae)
- Nodules (fibromas, fascial osteomas, fascial sarcomas, as in Fig. 122ab)

Fasciitis or *fibromatosis* of the fascia is manifested primarily in three ways:

3.7.1
Dupuytren's Contracture

Dupuytren's contracture (Fig. 95) is seen in the form of fibrotic changes of the palmar fascia. *Clinical*:

- Thickening and hardening of the superficial skin layers
- Pain-free, often symmetrical
- Restricted movement in the fingers (*contracture* mostly D3, Fig. 63)

3.7.2
Plantar Fasciitis

Plantar fasciitis is seen as a fibromatous inflammation in the plantar fascia (Fig. 98, CS 36), is often associated with new bone formation at the *calcaneus* and is described as

Calcaneopathia rheumatica in the form of *fibroostosis* or *fibroostitis* (called *calcaneal spur*) or *plantar fibromatosis* (identical to *Depuytren's* contracture of the hand).

Clinical:

- Severe pain in the heel and plantar region (with every step)
- Tenderness in the heels, mostly asymmetrical
- DD, rare conditions: metastasis, osteosarcoma, *Perthes* disease (*Osteodystrophia deformans*)

Radiological:

- *Calcaneal spur* (no correlation to the symptoms)/Fig. 108/

Certain diagnosis of *plantar fasciitis* is confirmed by MRI (Fig. 98, CS 36).

3.7.3
Diffuse Eosinophilic Fasciitis

Shulman's syndrome, special form of *SSc*:

- *Sclerodactyly* (thickening and hardening of the skin on the hands and feet) with tenderness and *contractures* (Chap. 9.1.4, Fig. 18)
- *Eosinophilia* on blood and skin-muscle biopsy
- *No Raynaud's* syndrome
- No evidence of organ involvement

3.8
Bursae (Bursitis)

This involves the bulging of tendon sheaths or joint capsules on account of periarticular bursitis with fluid retention. Large bursitides are defined as *cysts* and arthroceles or *tenosynovialitis*.

Clinical (Figs. 28, 42):

- Clearly definable, highly elastic swelling (subcutaneous or deep-seated) tenderness (in synovialitis, e.g., *RA*, Fig. 28; CS 10)
- ❖ Acute pain in the hollow of the knee and swelling in the lower leg (suspected perforation of Baker's cyst, refer to comments on Fig. 49 in Chap. 2, DD *acute thrombophlebitis* or calcareous deposits in *Bursitis subacromialis* and *Tendinitis calcarea*)
    - Pain-free variant (*Bursa olecrani*, Baker's cyst)

Radiological:

- Conventional X-ray
- Bone scan
- Ultrasound
- MRI

Most common localizations:

- Subacromial/subdeltoid (in *rotator cuff tendinitis* or *impingement syndrome*)
- Prepatellar (in *OA* with *synovitis*)
- Baker's cyst or popliteal cyst (in *RA* and other forms of arthritis)
- In olecranon (*RA, gout*)
- Wrists (*RA, sepsis*)
- Iliopsoas
- *Trochantor major* (in *OA* with *synovitis, RA, SpA*)

Most common causes:

- Inflammatory joint diseases (*RA, gout, pseudogout*)
- Degenerative joint diseases (*OA*)
- Local trauma or microtrauma
- Sepsis

3.9
Ligaments (Joint Instabilities, Deviations and Ruptures)

The ligament syndrome can be regarded as a consequence of inflammatory (Chap. 1.3, Figs. 42, 43, 70) and less often degenerative (Chap. 1.4) arthropathies, but also sport injuries. The underlying joint diseases could also cause joint instability due to cartilage (Fig. 26) and bone (Fig. 54) defects and may thus necessitate surgery (as in Fig. 122c). When ruling out such structural changes, any loosening or deviation in the joints must be viewed in relation to the ligaments.

Lead ligament symptoms:

- Abnormal mobility or instability of the joints and spinal column
- Uncertain gait
- Neurological and vascular damage with loosened ligaments in the cervical spine (due to *cervical arthritis* C1/C2) and lumbar regions, associated with *facet* syndrome (*pseudo-sciatica* syndrome)
- *Deviations* (e.g., ulnar deviation, *Genu vara*, and *valga*)
- *(Sub) luxations*
- Pain in the ligament system
- *Postural anomalies*, e.g., following arthrodesis of the hand (Fig. 122c) or ankle

Primary localizations:

- Hands (in *RA, CTD*)
- Shoulder (*adhesive capsulitis or idiopathic shoulder rigidity*)
- Cervical region (*cervical arthritis* C1/C2, Fig. 60)
- Lumbar region
- Knees
- Hips

The diagnosis should be investigated clinically and radiologically (CT, MRI in *cervical arthritis* and *facet* syndrome).

3.10
Bone Marrow

(See Chap. 9.9)

Here, arterial circulatory disorders or inflammation of the cellular structures of the bone are involved and are clinically manifested as follows:

3.10.1
Osteonecrosis

Osteonecrosis is considered to be the irreversible outcome of arterial circulatory disorders in the affected bone or bone segment, and can be asymmetrical or bilateral.

- Most common localizations:
  - Femoral head
  - Acetabulum (Fig. 121)
  - Medial femoral condyle (*Ahlbäck's* disease, *primary and secondary*)
  - Head of the humerus

Clinically there are no specific symptoms, only the features of the underlying disease (*OA* and/or *arthritis*); furthermore, consideration should be given to a differential diagnosis if the most common causes of *osteonecrosis* are present:

- Initially a discrepancy between the highly, almost always acute pain and/or restrictions in mobility (has been described as "bone crisis" in *Gaucher's* disease, for instance) and the relatively intact joint and bone compartments on conventional X-rays
- Long-term cortisone and immunosuppressive therapy, post-radiotherapy
- *SLE* (often bilateral) and inflammatory bowel diseases (*Crohn's* disease, *Colitis ulcerosa*)
- *Antiphospholipid* syndrome
- *Diabetic angiopathy*, hyperlipoproteinemia, *adiposis*

- *Gaucher's* disease (in the non-neuropathic form of lysosomal storage disease)
- *Alcoholism*

Diagnosis can be confirmed by

- Conventional X-rays and CT at an advanced stage (typical half-moon shaped subchondral translucency as far as destruction of the femoral head), DD *Paget's* disease (Chap. 3.11.3)
- Bone scan (cold zones) in early stages, DD *Paget's disease*
- MRI in early stages (dual band in T2 weighted image, Fig. 121, CS 44)

3.10.2
Osteitis

This is characterized by a noninfectious inflammation or irritative condition in the bones which can affect all bone structures. Unlike *osteomyelitis*, this is by no means a bacterial infection in the bone marrow, as could be the case in the event of open traumas, often following tooth extraction, *sepsis, TB,* or in immunosuppressed patients (*HIV*, post-chemotherapy). Nonbacterial changes in the bones have, to this extent, only been found upon introduction of MRI. Similar changes exist in the case of inflammation in the vertebral bodies (*spondylitis, spondylodiscitis*) or bones (*sacroiliitis, stress fractures*). Involvement of the bone marrow can be detected only by MRI (T1, T2 enhancement).

Otherwise *osteitis* has no specific clinical correlate and can, according to our data,[4] only be assured by MRI in the case of resistant *soft-tissue diseases* and, at that, equally as often with

- Mechanical and inflammatory factors in variable combinations with other forms of *STR* (Figs. 26, 102) or with
- *OA* with *synovitis* (hip/sacroiliac region).

3.11
Bone (Metabolic Osteopathies, Periostitis) and Cartilage (Relapsing Polychondritis)

Ossalgia (bone pain) is one of the most common symptoms, but does not necessarily indicate bone involvement; infections and metabolic, neoplastic, neurological aspects should be taken into account. The bone metabolism disorders presented here are manifested as *osteoporosis, osteomalacia, Ostitis deformans,* and *hypertrophic osteoarthropathy* as well as *secondarily* in endocrinological (*hyperparathyroidism*) and metabolic (*Fabry's* and *Gaucher's* disease could arise with agonizing pain in the extremities) diseases (*Relapsing polychondritis* see Chap. 9.8).

3.11.1
Osteoporosis

Lead symptoms (Figs. 125–127, CS 46) (one of the most common, widespread diseases):

- Bone pain, possibly the first signs (broad DD necessary): *plasmocytoma, bone tumor,* or *metastasis*
- Bone fractures, also *stress fractures* (Fig. 54): "gradual" (in vertebrae) and resulting from falls, often in older adults regardless of the degree of trauma and with acute neurological symptoms
- Diminished height (sintering)
- *Osteopenia* or *osteoporosis* in bone density measurement (by DEXA, a recommendation which at present applies only to women)
  - Normal bone density: T-score +/−1 standard deviations from mean of *peak bone mass*
  - *Osteopenia*: T-score −1 to −2.5 from the above mentioned standard deviations
  - *Osteoporosis*: T-score more than −2.5 from the above mentioned standard deviations
- Deformation of axial skeleton (hunched back, scoliosis)
- Most common localizations for bone fractures:
  - Spine (thoracal and lumbal, most often Th7-L1)
  - Hip, ribs, femoral neck, distal radius

Forms of *osteoporosis*:

- *Primary*
  - Postmenopausal women (menopausal type I *osteoporosis*)
  - Advanced age over 75 years, associated with dramatic increase in the incidence of bone fractures (senile, type II *osteoporosis*)
  - *Secondary*
    - Glucocorticoid-induced, type III *osteoporosis* (CS 46)
    - Endocrinopathies (*Cushing's, hyperparathyroidism, hyperthyroidism,* estrogen/testosterone deficiency, *diabetes mellitus* → Chap. 1.5.2)
- Local *osteoporosis (RA, SpA, Sjögren's* and *Sudeck's* syndrome, radiotherapy, *vasculitis,* and *plasmocytoma*)
- Preclinical *osteoporosis* (*no bone fractures* at the time of measurement)
- Manifest (advanced) *osteoporosis* (known *bone fractures* also "silent")

Predisposing factors:

- Race (Caucasians and Asians affected much more often than those with colored skin)
- Limited mobility
- Lack of sun exposure

3.11.2
Osteomalacia

A metabolic disorder of skeletal mineralization caused by vitamin D deficiency or resistance secondary *hyperparathyroidism* (Chap. 1.5.2).

Lead symptoms:

- *Bone pain*, diffuse (caused by *osteoporosis* and possibly fractures)
- Flexion deformities and skeletal deformity
- Growth inhibition (*rachitis*)
- Increased stress fractures
- *Myasthenia* of proximal extremities
- Hypotension
- *Elevated alkaline phosphatase* in the serum (also in *Paget's* disease)
- *Hypocalcemia* and *phosphate deficiency* (as with *hypoparathyroidism*)
- *Radiological*: decalcified zones

Most common localizations: Metaphyses of the long hollow bones, spinal column, ribs, pelvis, and femoral neck (fractures).

Predisposing factors:

- Reduced vitamin D supply from:
  - Diet
  - Lack of sun (veiled women)
  - Gastrectomy
  - Celiac sprue
  - *Scleroderma* with intestinal involvement
- Renal diseases (tubular and glomerular)
- *Hyperparathyroidism*

3.11.3
Ostitis Deformans (Paget's Disease)

This disease is a form of genetically induced *osteopathy* (increased incidence in some countries and families), characterized by focal disorganization of the bone architecture (uncoordinated combination of osteolytic and osteosclerotic changes) and mechanical inferiority of the bone.

Lead symptoms:

- Bone, joint, and muscle pain (heels, thoracic, and lumber spine syndrome)
- *Secondary OA*

- Deformities ("saber tibia" in the form of O-legs, thoracic kyphosis)
- Increased stress fractures
- Cranial enlargement with subsequent
  - Cranial nerve paralysis (loss of hearing, loss of vision)
- Bottleneck syndromes (Chap. 3.12.1) on account of increased bone formation
- *Elevated serum alkaline phosphatase* (with normal Ca^2+ and liver enzymes) is a marker of osteoblatic activity and indicator of skeletal extent and activity
- Most patients are asymptomatic despite the remarkable appearance on X-ray and bone scan
  X-ray:
  - Combined pattern of *osteolytic* (*osteoporosis circumscripta* mit areas of sharply demarcated radiolucency) and *osteoblastic* or *osteosclerotic* (thickening of cortical structures, osteosclerosis in vertebrae) regions; such a pattern also with metastases and *plasmocytoma*
  - Cysts and deformities
- Bone scan:
  - Enhancement upon increased bone metabolism
  - Determination of number of affected bones and extent of the involvement

Most common localizations: pelvis, skull, lumbar and thoracic spine, femur, cranium, tibia.

3.11.4
Hypertrophic Osteoarthropathy (Drumstick Fingers)

This syndrome is characterized by periostal bony formations on the long, hollow bones and the skin/nails of the distal extremities, developing as *primary* (hereditary) or *secondary* (pulmonary, cardiac diseases with hypoxia, *tumors, PsA*, chronic infections/*Endocarditis lenta*/or intestinal diseases).

Lead symptoms (Fig. 88):

- Drumstick fingers and hourglass nails on the hands and feet
- Bone pain
- Periostal and periarticular pain with noninflammatory effusion
- Skin thickening
- Cyanotic cardiac and pulmonary diseases
- Malignant tumors/metastases
- *Radiological*:
  - *Periostal* reaction, also in long hollow bones (DD *PsA*)
  - *Acroosteolysis* in the fingers

- Bone scan:
  - Enhancement in periosteum of the long bones with determination of
  - Number of affected bones
  - Extent of involvement

Most common localizations: fingers, toes, tibia
  Predisposing factors: genetic (increased incidence in certain countries and families)

3.11.5
Periostitis

Periostitis is to be regarded as a component of the bundle of *STR*, namely of the muscle–tendon–ligament apparatus with periosteal new bone formation, among *mechanical* joint and spinal diseases and the *inflammatory*:

- Rheumatic (e.g., *SpA, PAN, MPA, SAPHO*-syndrome)
- Other diseases (sarcoidose, Crohn's)
- Infections (Syphilis, HIV)
- Malignancy (secondary hypertrophic osteoarthropathy)

The disease can be suspected in the event of severe, persistent, therapy-resistant, local pressure and percussion pain (mostly in the spine and long bones and calcaneal). In one of our cases, such a suspicion was confirmed in an *HIV* positive patient by MRI of the *tibia*.

3.11.6
Relapsing Polychondritis

Rare inflammatory autoimmune disease or a condition characterized as auricular *chondritis* (spares the earlobe, Fig. 29). There was widespread involvement of cartilage tissue and tissues rich in proteoglycans, such as the eyes and heart valves. Local auricular cartilage infestation is commonly seen. In this case a cartilage biopsy, a traumatic event, is not essential for making a diagnosis (see comment on Fig 29, *RCS*, Chap. 2). These local forms of *auricular chondritis*, accompanied by severe pain symptoms, respond well to glucocorticoids.

In other cases *relapsing polychondritis* exhibited a wide range of broad potential targets (Chap. 9.8):

- Inflammatory changes in the cartilage (ears, nose with subsequent deformity, rarely the tracheal cartilage)
- Often associated with organ involvement (skin, joints, eyes, cochlear or vestibular disorders, cardiovascular syndrome, CNS and kidneys)

In our case (Fig. 29) symmetrical *auricular chondritis* was associated with *RA*-like polyarthritis of the MCP and PIP joints, which, incidentally, developed 2 months later. The connection of the two syndromes simply illustrates the course of the disease.

3.11.7
Perichondritis or Synchondrosis Manubriosternalis

Perichondritis is also characterized by stable, resistant (pressure) pain symptoms in the sternum, developing post-sternotomy after cardiac surgery (Fig. 61, CS 21). Both syndromes are diagnosed by means of MRI examination.

3.11.8
Osteochondromatosis or Chondroblastoma

A benign disease which results in metaplastic restructuring of the synovial tissue into cartilage and bony tissue, possibly leading to the formation of loose bodies in the joints or benign tumors in the bones (*enchondroma* as in Fig. 36b).

- Most often localized in the large joints (elbows, knees, hips), rarely the skull
- Diagnosis is obtained with X-ray or MRI, by ascertaining loose bodies in the joints or ossified islands of cartilage

---

3.12
Nerves

Nerve involvement (in *CTD* and *vasculitis* → Chap. 9.7) is considered in the event of:

- *Pain*, mostly at night, radiating on account of radicular innervation
- *Sensibility disorders* (paresthesias, abnormal sensations, hypoesthesias, hyperalgesias, pareses, weakened reflexes)
- *Motoric disorders, muscular atrophies*
- The symptoms can be provoked by certain mechanical factors (coughing, sneezing, flexion, extension, percussion, and compression)

Such symptoms are seen, depending on the root affected, along the length of the related dermatomes and myotomes in the following circumstances:

3.12.1
Root Compression Syndrome

Radiculopathies are characterized by radicular pain with sensory and/or motor, but also medullary and vascular deficits in the case of degenerative and inflammatory *spine* diseases:

- Life-threatening *medullary* and *vascular compression* syndrome in *RA, SpA*, and *spine* fractures, arising from *osteoporosis* (Fig. 126, CS 46)
- *Pseudo-sciatica* syndromes or "facet pain" (mostly in the case of *spondylarthrosis* and *tendomyosis*), induced by neural and vascular irritation of the muscles, tendons, and ligaments:
  - Local pain with radiation and sensory deficits
  - No motor deficits
  - No alleviation of pain from a change in posture
- *Plexus* syndrome is neurological in nature; e.g., brachial plexopathy can result from many causes (traumatic, infectious, diabetes, tumor, degenerative etiology, or median sternotomy done for cardiac surgery)
- *Bottleneck* syndrome (*compression* syndrome in the peripheral nerves)
  The most common bottleneck syndromes in peripheral nerves:
  - *Carpal tunnel* syndrome (distal median nerve)
  - *Loge de Guyon* syndrome (distal ulnar nerve) (Fig. 122, CS 45)
  - *Sulcus ulnaris* syndrome (proximal ulnar nerve)
  - *Thoracic outlet* syndrome (cervicobrachial plexus)
  - *Tarsal tunnel* syndrome (distal tibial nerve)
  - *Morton's* neuralgia (interdigital nerves)
  - *Meralgia paresthetica* (compression of the lateral femoral cutaneous nerve)

3.12.2
Neuropathies

- *Polyneuropathies* (axonal in *CTD, vasculitis*, demyelinating in *diabetes mellitus, alcohol*)
- *Mononeuropathy multiplex* or *mononeuritis simplex* in systemic *vasculitis, RA, borreliosis*, and *sarcoidosis* (facial palsy) (See Chap. 9.7)

Neurophysiological examinations (electromyography and electroneurography) are necessary in order to assess the level, character (axonal or demyelinating), floridity, and severity of nerve damage and differentiate from *pseudoradicular pain* syndromes, respectively.

3.13
Periarticular Structures (Periarthropathies)

Periarticular disorders or *periarthropathy humeroscapularis* (*PHS*) are characterized by inflammatory and/or degenerative changes in the periarticular structures (bursa, tendon, capsule). In the most common form, *tendinitis of the rotator cuff* (*RCT*), such changes are highly complex and polydimensional, affecting the ligaments and tendons (mostly the *supraspinatus* and *biceps* tendon) with partial or full rupture, fascia, tendon attachments, bursae with calcium deposits (acute *crystal bursitis* and *calcific tendinitis* as a correlate to severe pain), muscles and fascia with fibrosis of the joint capsule (*adhesive capsulitis*) in varying combinations and of varying pronouncements. For this reason *periarticular disorders* present in various clinical forms with different names, i.e., *impingement* syndrome (see Chap. 4.1), fibrosis of the shoulder capsule, *cuff syndrome, subacromial bursitis*:

PHS is diagnosed on the basis of

- *Clinical* symptoms (CS 39, Fig. 106):
  - Diffuse or localized pain on movement with radiation, pressure, run-in, nocturnal pain
  - Painful and passive movement restrictions, relieving posture
  - *Muscular atrophy* and *paresis*
  - *Shoulder-hand* syndrome is characterized by *PHS ankylosans* and *Sudeck's* dystrophy of the hand
- *Radiology*
  - Calcium deposits in the rotator cuff
  - *Bursitis calcarea* (*Bursitis subacromialis*)
- Sonogram and MRI, in particular, confirm the diagnosis
- Negative imaging does not rule out the diagnosis
- Positive radiological changes are not sufficient on their own (without clinical findings)

Most common localizations for *periarthropathies*

- Shoulder *PHS* appears in the following clinical forms:
  - Acute (synonym: tendinitis/*Tendinosis calcarea, PHS calcificans*)
  - *Tendopathia simplex* (supraspinatus, biceps longus, biceps brevis)
  - Adhesive (*adhesive capsulitis*)
  - *Frozen shoulder* (restriction of active and passive movement of the shoulder due to synovitis and reactive capsular fibrose)
  - *Pseudoparetica* (acute development of "paralysis" of the arm due to ruptured rotator cuff)
  - *Ankylosans* (increasing rigidity, could be self-limiting)
  - With reflex dystrophy (*shoulder-hand* syndrome, *osteitis, CRP* elevation)
- Hips *periarthritis coxae*
- Knees *periarthritis genu*

Primary degenerative diseases of the periarticular structures are most frequently involved, namely tendons, joint capsules, and calcium deposits, spontaneous and traumatic ruptures of the tendons. All such changes are summarized under the generic term of *PHS. Rotator cuff disorders* as a component of the *PHS* represent a spectrum of conditions, including inflammation, partial- or full-thickness tears, and cuff tear arthropathy.

Sonogram and MRI, in particular, confirm the diagnosis of *PHS*

Regional Arthrological and Musculoskeletal Syndromes

4

4.1
Shoulder

In the case of shoulder pain, the following etiologies should be considered primarily:

- *Polymyalgia rheumatica* (CS 52), most bilateral aching in shoulder and/or pelvic girdle (among patients over 50 years of age)
- *Tendomyosis* (muscle strain of the noninflammatory origin) → Chap. 3.4
- *Articular cause*:
  - *Inflammatory shoulder* pain (*cervical arthritis, shoulder arthritis* in *RA, AS*/ Fig. 60/, crystal arthropathy, can involve the glenohumeral, sternoclavicular, or acromioclavicular joints)
  - *Degenerative arthritis* or *OA* (*Arthrosis acromioclavicularis*, subacromial impingement with degenerative tendopathy)
- *Periarticular disorders:*
  - *Rotator cuff tendinitis/insertion tendopathy* (*supraspinatus, subscapularis muscles, bicipital*); the pathology ranging from tendinitis and bursitis to partial tearing, to complete tear in one or more of the tendons (long biceps tendon, supraspinatus tendon)/Fig. 106/
  - *Adhesive capsulitis* and *frozen shoulder*associated with capsular adhesion and synovitis, are syndrome, in which both active and pasive motion is lost because of soft-tissue contracture
  - *Bursitis (Bursa subacromialis et subdeltoidea)*/Fig. 106/,
  - *Impingement* syndrome (*other perspective* on the periarticular disorders, see Chap. 3.13):
    - Classical (*external*) *impingement* to be caused by compression of the subacromial bursa, long head of the biceps tendon and rotator cuff by the coracoacromial arch
    - *Internal* due to *impingement* of the soft tissue, including the rotator cuff, joint capsule of the posterosuperior part of the glenoid

E. Benenson, *Rheumatology*, Symptoms and Syndromes
DOI: 10.1007/978-1-84996-462-3_4, © Springer-Verlag London Limited 2011

- *Nerve disorders:*
  - *Cervicobrachial* syndrome, pseudo-radicular or radicular spine/*sciatica*/syndrome (CS 63) in cervical *spondylosis* with subacute radiculopathy (much more common) and myelopathy (the most commonly involved discs are C5–6 and C6–7)
  - *Brachial plexopathy* is a neurogenic cause of severe shoulder pain (Chap. 3.12.1)
  - *Neuropathy (subscapularis, axillaris nerves,* etc.) → Chap. 3.12.2

Accentuated problems with the shoulder are, in certain diseases, termed as *diabetic shoulder* or *frozen shoulder.* In known cases of noninflammatory *OA* of the shoulder and acromioclavicular joints, *RA* or *SpA*, pain in the shoulder should be given greater attention.

A *new* pain pattern (with pain and stiffness in the neck) and *new* constellations (disproportionately severe signs of inflammation with minimally active *RA* are indicative of another disease, namely, *polymyalgia rheumatica,* CS 52).

For the purposes of differentiation, it must be ascertained whether the shoulder pain is *symmetrical (polymyalgia rheumatica)* or *asymmetrical (coronary artery disease, lung tumors).*

When *initially* attempting to rule out these diseases, imaging, primarily MRI, should be instigated, particularly with a view to therapy (Figs. 106, 107), prognosis, and if necessary, orthopedic treatment.

In the event of *subacromial impingement,* for instance, consideration is to be given to subacromial decompression, synovectomy, and partial clavicular resection.

Orthopedic specialists should, if the pain is severe and movement restricted in the shoulders, investigate the following *conditions, which may require surgery*:

- Narrowing of the claviculoacromial space
- Chronic, especially *pannus-like synovitis*
- *Septic arthritis* (following infiltration therapy)
- *Tendinosis calcarea* (shock wave therapy, if necessary)
- *Aseptic necrosis*
- Bone and tendon *ruptures*
- *Destructive* inflammatory and degenerative *arthriti0073*

4.2
Chest Wall and Anterior Chest Wall Syndrome

(Such is the term for painful swelling and thickening of the sternoclavicular regions and breast) should be differentiated.

Diagnostic concept for *chest pain* and discomfort:

- Exclusion of other diseases (cardiac, pulmonary, vascular, gastrointestinal, cervical disk disease, vertebral and rib fractures, neuralgia, particularly *Herpes zoster,* tumors)
- Exclusion of the *OA* of the thorax spine as well as compression of the brachial plexus by a cervical rib or by spasm of the scalenus muscle

- Screening for *primary* inflammatory musculoskeletal diseases (e.g., *RA*, *AS* with *spondylodiscitis*/CS 17/, *antiphospholipid* syndrome with pulmonary embolism (possibly in patients with CS 3, 6), *Takayasu's arteritis* (CS 21), *coronaritis* with myocardial infarctions in *vasculitis* (CS 21, 26, Figs. 74, 77) and *CTD* (*SLE*, *SSc*)
- A bone scan should be taken to check for local or systemic changes. Then the next step can be taken:
- If there are unexplained local changes, a conventional X-ray and MRI should be performed

The *localization* of the chest pain is of pivotal importance to the diagnosis.

4.2.1
Sternoclavicular (Tietze, SAPHO Syndrome, Costochondritis, and Arthritis)

Clinically this is mostly seen as a painful, hard swelling (mostly asymmetrical) of the costal cartilage, primarily of the first joint (Fig. 69), taking the form of

- *Tietze's* syndrome (*primary* disease resulting from *osteochondrosis* of the sternocostal joints or *arthritis* of the same joints associated with, e.g., *PsA*, CS 23 or *acne*)
  - *Chondrocostal precordial* syndrome is manifested as *angina pectoris* – similar left-sided precordial pain when resting, with pressure points on the 2nd to 4th left sternocostal joints
  - *Costochondritis/enthesitis* is manifested by painful costochondral articulations (tends to affect the other joints) without swelling, associated with *RA*, *SpA*, *ReA*, and *sarcoidosis*
- *SAPHO* syndrome comprises the following syndromes:
  - *S* = synovitis (Fig. 68) or, and not uncommonly, *dactylitis* (Figs. 65ab)
  - *A* = acne (cf. comments on Figs. 65ab)
  - *P* = pustulosis (Figs. 110, 111a, 129b)
  - *H* = hyperostosis (Fig. 118)
  - *O* = osteitis (as in Figs. 102, 108, 121)
- *Arthritis* of the shoulder or spine associated with *RA* or *SpA*
- *Tendomyopathy* (sternocostal *tender points* in *fibromyalgia*)
- *Myositis* (PM/DM, sarcoidosis)

4.2.2
Parasternal

- *Enthesiopathy* associated with *SpA* (sternocostal)
- *Arthritis* associated with *RA* or *SpA*
- *Mastitis*, ANA-positive as an early sign of SLE with single organ manifestation (CS 38)
- Mastodynia

4.2.3
Band-like

(On deep inspiration, coughing):

- *Arthritis* of costotransversal and costovertebral joints
- *Herpes zoster*
- Slipping rib syndrome, which usually involves the tenth rib
- Intercostal muscle cramps
- Pleurisy, pleuritis (in CTD, RA, Still's, see Chap. 10.4.2)

4.2.4
Sternal Pain

- *Synchondrosis manubriosternalis* (status post thoracotomy, CS 21)
- Xiphoidalgia
- Pericarditis (Chap. 10.4.1)

4.2.5
Thoracic Rigidity

(In *SSc*/CS 19/ and *SpA*).

4.3
Elbows

This is one of the most commonly affected regions.
   Clinical:

- (Pressure) pain, also with certain movements (gripping, turning and rotating)
- Stiffness and restricted movement (also when closing the fist and in the cervical spine region)
- Disfiguration, deformities, contractures
- Node formation (*rheumatoid nodules, tophi* or *calcinoses*)

Background:
   Articular diseases (Chap. 1) predominantly in:

- Monoarthritic attacks
  - *(Non)-inflammatory OA*
  - *Bacterial arthritis, SpA*
  - *Arthropathies* (neuropathic, hemophilia, among others)
  - *(Sub)-luxations* of the radial head

- Polyarthritic attacks
  - *RA*
  - *SpA* (possibly all forms)
  - *(Pseudo) gout arthritis*
- Soft-tissue conditions (*insertion tendinitis* → Chap. 3.6.1)
  - *Epicondylitis radialis*, lateral ("tennis elbow")
  - *Epicondylitis ulnaris*, medial ("golfer's elbow")
  - *Tendinitis* of musculotendinous insertion of biceps
- Ulnar neuropathy and
- Nerve entrapment

Such changes occur most often within the context of

- *Localized* (Chap. 3.4) or *generalized* (Chap. 3.5) tendomyopathy
- *cervical spine* syndrome (Chap. 2.1.1)
- *Bursitis olecrani* possibly with nodules (in *RA*, *gout* arthritis, burdens: "student's elbow" and sport injuries)
- *Bone and bone marrow diseases* (Chaps. 3.10 and 3.11)
  - *Chondrocalcinosis*
  - *Osteomalacia*
  - *Fractures*
  - *Epiphyseal necrosis*

Stiffness is expressed as total extension deficits (due to *inflammatory arthritis*, e.g., in *SpA*, *RA* among others) or as *contractures*, and should be regarded in combination with *deformities*, if applicable, as a consequence of chronic fibrosing-ankylosing *arthritis* (in *RA*, *PsA*, *gout*, and *Jaccoud's* arthropathy with *CTD*, Fig. 70). Sonogram and MRI, in particular, can confirm the diagnosis.

4.4
Wrists

The (sub) acute functional deficit of the wrists (due to pain) is associated with:

- *Inflammatory arthritis*, mostly *RA*, *crystal*-associerte arthritis, *septic* arthritis (Fig. 115)
- *Aseptic necrosis*, osteolysis of the bone in *RA* or of unknown etiology, as in Fig. 34; *Kienbock's* disease (avascular necrosis of the lunate bone)
- *Bone destruction* (Figs. 51, 54, 122 ac) and fractures
- *Enthesiopathy* (periarthritis, e.g., *Styloiditis radii*), bursitis (Fig. 42)
- *Triangular disc* syndrome (in traumatic, degenerative and inflammatory injury to the fibrous cartilage on the outer side of the wrist, "the vertebral disc in the wrist")

(Sub) acute functional deficit in the fingers often occurs at the level of the wrist. For that are, thereby, responsible:

- Spontaneous *ruptures* of the extensor and flexor tendons (as in Fig. 42)
- *Tenosynovitis* of the wrist
- *Ganglion*
- *Compression* syndrome in form of *radial nerve palsy* (CS 45)
- *Subluxations* and ulnar *deviations* (Fig. 70)
- Massive *rheumatoid nodules* (Figs. 122ab)

Most common localizations:

- Extensor tendons of 5th and 4th fingers (Figs. 70, 95)
- Flexor tendons of 1st, 2nd, and 5th fingers (Fig. 42).

The *most common causes* are

- *RA*
- *OA* of the wrist
- Radial *fractures*
- Status post *surgery*

Imaging (sonogram, X-ray, MRI) can confirm the diagnosis.

4.5
Hands

Here it is of particular importance to identify a morphological substrate of the pain and swelling in the hand. In principle, all structures could be affected (Chaps. 1.5, 9.2.3):

- *Joints and periarticular structures* in
  - *Inflammatory OA, Heberden's*, and *Bouchard's* (Figs. 4, 8, 81, 128ab)
  - *RA* (Figs. 3, 9ab, 28, 35, 40, 42, 49, 51, 58, 59, 64, 80, 104, 129 ac)
  - *PsA* (Figs. 68, 110), *gout* (Figs. 13, 130ab), and other forms of *arthritis* (Fig. 21)
  - *Arthropathy* (Fig. 19)
  - *CTD: SSc* (Figs. 18, 130c), *CREST* (Fig. 89), *MCTD* (Figs. 7, 70), *SLE* (Fig. 128c)
  - *Osteolysis* syndrome (etiologically unexplained bone resorption/*vanishing bone disease*/with "indifferent" bone defects, as in Fig. 34)
- *Tendons and tendon sheaths* (*tendinitis, trigger finger*)/Fig. 63/
- *Fasciae* (*Dupuytren's, fasciitis*), mostly combined with *tendinitis* (Fig. 95) or *volar flexor tenosynovitis* (Fig. 104 right)
- *Bones* (*erosive destructive arthritis, aseptic necrosis*)
- *Nerves* (*compression* syndrome/Fig. 122/, *Sudeck's* syndrome (such as in Fig. 66), *polyneuropathy, carpal tunnel* syndrome

- *Vascular* (*Raynaud's* syndrome, *vasculitis*, Figs. 14, 47, 52, 66)
    - *Palmar erythema* in *RA* (Fig. 100), liver, *graft-versus-host* diseases
- *Psychogenic factors* (*psychogenic rheumatism* or *somatogenic pain* syndrome/CS 57, 61/, has recently been included as the diagnosis "symptoms of pain with somatic and psychological factors" *ICD*-10 (*International Classification of Diseases*) in the chapter "Somatoform Disorders."
- *Angioedema*, hereditary (an early symptom in one of our patients)
- *Fabry's* disease (agonizing pain in the hands and feet as an early symptom)
- Diabetic *hand* syndrome; *scleroderma-like syndrome*, *fat fingers* and *contractures*, with no acral necrosis (Fig. 130a)

Sonogram and MRI, in particular, can confirm the diagnosis. The *explanations* to all Figs. and all CS are presented in *RCS*, Chap. 2, and the solutions as well as *diagnoses* in the *RCS*, Appendix.

4.6
Changes in the Fingers and Toes

Involvement of these structures is of enormous significance to the diagnostic process, and since they are highly specific, an assured diagnosis of one disease or at least one condition is possible (Figs. 128–130, visual diagnostics).

4.6.1
Deformities in the Fingers and Toes

Such changes are associated with over-extension and ruptures of the extensor apparatus, contractures of the musculature, *arthritis*, and/or *OA*. They include:

- *Arthritis*, floride or proliferative: *acute gout* (Fig. 13), *SpA* (Figs. 21, 24), *RA* (Figs. 28, 35), also because of *rheumatoid nodules* (Fig. 104), *OA* (Fig. 128a)
- *Extensor deficits of the proximal interphalangeal joints* (Figs. 5, 40, 42, 70, 81, 104); etiology: *RA*, degenerative or traumatic *rupture* of the extensor tendons
- *Deformities of the basilar thumb* (simultaneous imaging/CS 1/: Figs. 5, 9a/pre-op/, 9b/post-op/; Figs. 35, 58; compare against MCP 1 in Figs. 22 and 59); etiology: *RA*, *basilar thumb* and nodal (DIP and PIP) *OA*
- *Tenosynovitis* of extensore tendons (Fig. 42) in *RA*, and palmar
- *De Quervain's tenosynovitis* (Fig. 5, this patient has severe pain with thumb extension and abduction and palpable crepitation of the first dorsal extensor compartment)
- *Palmar subluxation of the fingers* (Figs. 42 and 104) in *RA*
- *Contractures* (Figs. 70, 80, 95, 130a) or *claw hand* (Figs. 18, 19, 62) in *RA*, nodal *OA*, *polyneuropathy, tetraparesis*
- *Ulnar deviation* of the fingers (Fig. 42) in *RA*, other forms of *destructive arthritis*, *cerebral paresis*, and rupture of the deep flexor tendon

- *Fixed malpositioning* of the toe joints in *RA* (Fig. 43), *PsA*, *OA*
- *Hallux valgus*: genetically induced, *OA* of the first metatarsophalangeal joint
- *Vascular* causes of pain (Chap. 9.2)

4.6.2
Swelling of the Fingers and Hands ("Puffy Fingers")

in:

- *SSs* (initial stage)/Fig. 130c/
- *Diabetes mellitus* (Fig. 130a)
- *Septic arthritis* (Fig. 115)
- *Fibromyalgia* (CS 57, 61)
- *Mixed CTD* (Fig. 7)
- *Tenobursitis* of the wrists in *RA* (Figs. 42, 80, 104)
- *RS3PE* syndrome (remitting seronegative symmetrical synovitis with pitting edema)
- *Hypothyroidism*
- *Allergy*
- *Median nerve entrapment* syndrome (often accompanying *RA*)
- *Unknown origin* (Fig. 66)

4.6.3
Dactylitis

("sausage finger," "sausage toe," Figs.15a, 41, 65ab)

- "Hot-spot" involvement (three-way joint involvement of a finger or toe)/Fig. 49b, second left digit; Fig. 64, third left digit/
    - *PsA*
    - *ReA*
    - *SAPHO*
    - *Acne*-induced *arthritis*
- Swelling of the entire soft tissue of a finger or toe
    - *Inflammatory OA, Heberden's,* and *Bouchard's* (Figs. 4, 81, 128a)
    - *Gout arthritis* (Fig. 13, e.g., *podagra*)
    - *Borreliosis*

4.6.4
Drumstick Fingers and Hour-Glass Nails

in:

- *Hypertrophic osteoarthropathy* (Chap. 3.11.4)
- *PsA* (Fig. 88)

4.7
Foot, Heel

4.7.1
Calcaneopathy

The *most significant localizations* are:

- *Hind foot pain* is most often caused by *tendinitis* (CS 37, Fig. 102), *arthritis* and *OA* of the tarsal joints, e.g., due to flat foot
- *Heel pain* is characterized by calcaneal spur (*fibroostitis*, Fig. 108), *plantar fasciitis* (Fig. 98), with (Fig. 102) or without (Fig. 103) *osteitis*
- *Achillodynia* should initially be regarded as linked to *tendinitis* or *Bursitis subachillea*, the nature of which can be mechanical (sport injuries) as often as inflammatory (SpA, RA). *Achillodynia*, with no MRI confirmation of a morphological substrate, could have an *underlying psychosomatic cause*

4.7.2
Metatarsalgia

(Pain of the midfoot):

- *Arthropathy* (*arthritis, SpA*)
- *Tendopathy* and *fasciitis*
- *Panniculitis* (Fig. 6)
- *Periostitis, plantar bursitis*
- *Plantar fibromatosis* (identical to Depuytren's contracture of the hand)
- *Fatigue* or *stress fracture*
- "Localized" *vasculitis* (Fig. 2)
- *Compartment* syndrome (from muscle overload due to sport, fracture, plaster cast)

4.7.3
Pain in the Toes

(Often with swelling) See Chap. 4.6:

- *MTP arthritis*, symmetrical or more rarely asymmetrical (Fig. 24) should be ascribed to *SpA* or *oligo-/monoarthritis, HLA-B27 positive* (CS 8) or to *PsA* (Fig. 15a)
- Initial symptoms of *RA* in the form of *dactylitis*, very typical, especially MTP 5 (Fig. 41, CS 14), which, with the suspicion of a *tumor* required surgery
- *Oligo-/mono-MTP arthritides* are possibly consistent with inflammatory *OA* or *ReA* and *SpA*, respectively
- *MTP 1 deformity* (a) symmetrical, is mostly degenerative by nature (*Arthrosis valgus*). Swelling should be interpreted within the context of inflammatory *OA* or *gout arthritis* (Fig. 130b)

- *Dactylitis* of the first toe should be seen as an indicator of *gout arthritis* (even in a 10-year-old girl, CS 55), but also of *PsA* without or with *osteitis* (Fig. 15a) or *acne-arthropathy* (Figs. 65ab), or *borreliosis*
- *Raynaud's* syndrome
- *Foot deformities* (e.g., flat-splayed feet)
- *Stress* fractures
- *Morton's neuralgia* (in the intermetatarsal spaces).

Imaging (sonogram, X-ray, MRI) can confirm the diagnosis

4.8
Calf Pain

(Acute occurrence often implies an *emergency situation*):

4.8.1
Phlebothrombosis or Thrombophlebitis

Phlebothrombosis of the deep branches of the *V. femoralis* should be ruled out, above all, in the case of such symptoms (if necessary with angiological consultation or hospitalization)

4.8.2
Rupture of Baker's Cyst

Rupture of Baker's cyst is a rare, but relatively dramatic (acute, severe pain "like the stab of a knife" (see explanations on Fig. 49) incident with an enlargement of the calf circumference.

4.8.3
Muscle Rupture

(From physical overexertion, our own observation in a female marathon runner on the circuit)

4.8.4
Erythema Nodosum

Erythema nodosum (Fig. 109) and other forms of *panniculitis* (Chaps. 3.2.1, 9.4.1)

4.9
Ankles

Clinically, it is important to distinguish:

- *Intra-articular* pain with dorsiflexion and plantar flexion of the foot
- *Extra-articular pain:* posterior medial and lateral, anterior lateral

4.9.1
(Sub) Acute and Chronic Pain

- Within the context of *RA, SpA, HLA-B27*-associated *arthritis* (often in *Yersinia* infection and *SpA*), *crystal-induced,* and *septic* arthritis
- *Acute sarcoidosis* (*Löfgren's* syndrome), refer also to morphologically confirmed skin lesions (Figs. 83, 90):
  - *Arthritis* (clinical, in actual fact *periarthritis*)
  - *Erythema nodosum* (Fig. 109)
  - *Bihilar lymphadenopathy* (Fig. 91)
- *Inflammatory OA*, subtalar, talonavicular (on radiological diagnosis)
- *Neuropathic arthropathy* with severe *OA* at *diabetes mellitus*
- *Arthropathy* (*hemochromatosis*, CS 50)
- *Monoarthritis* of the right ankle – the clinical manifestation of a *bone tumor* or *stress fracture* (Fig. 54)
- Lateral pre-malleolar *bursitis* (at plantar-flexed position of the foot)
- *Malpositioning* (e.g., following arthrodesis or ankylosis)
- *Compression* syndrome (tarsal tunnel, posterior talar impingement)

4.9.2
Acute Swelling around the Ankle (Periarticular)

- *Insertion tendopathies* (*achilles tendinitis*, CS 65)
- *Tendinitis* posterior tibial (posterior medial ankle pain, Fig. 102, MRI))
- *Painful soft-tissue edema*, confirmed by MRI (in female patient with *sacroiliitis*)
- *Panniculitis* (Figs. 6 and 71)

4.10
Knees

Varying degrees and combinations of monoarticular pain, instability and effusions, in light of their etiology (sport injuries, arthritis and/or OA), are of great significance to further rheumatological and orthopedic diagnostic procedures:

4.10.1
(Sub) Acute Pain

(Sub) acute pain and joint blockade, particullarly, with articular effusion:

- Torn meniscus, most often medial, *chondromalacia* (Figs. 25, 26)
- Meniscal injuries, rupture of cruciate ligament, most often anterior
- Quadriceps tendon rupture (following trauma, the patient can no longer actively extend the knee; visible indentation above the patella)
- *Patellar tendinosis (*"jumper's knee"*)*; by chronic overload of the knee extensor apparatus, tenderness of the patellar tendon with the knee in full extension
- Fat pad impingement syndrome (*Hoffa's* disease), acute or chronic impingement of the intrapattelar fat-pad between the patella and femur
- *Tendinitis* and *peritendinitis* of the quadriceps tendon. *Cave*: cortisone may *never* be injected directly into the tendon (only *peritendinous* injection)
- *Arthritis* in *RA, PsA, crystal-induced, SLE, gonorrhea*
- *Septic arthritis* (iatrogenic, following puncture, TNF therapy)
- *Arterial occlusion* (absent pulses with loss of sensation and strength), Fig. 132.
- *Intermittent hydrarthrosis* (episodic attacks of synovitis occur usually in one knee at a time)
- *Pigmented villonodular synovitis* (typically develops in the knee)

4.10.2
Chronic Pain

- *Inflammatory OA*
- Retropatellar *OA*
- *Chondromalacia* patellae
- *Chondrocalcinosis*
- Meniscal lesions
- Cruciate ligament lesions
- *Enthesiopathies* (attachment tendinitis), periarthropathies, trigger points, intra-articular ganglia
- *Enthesitis* around the knee, relatively common lesions associated with *SpA*
- *Iliotibial band* syndrome (pain that radiates down the lateral thigh to the tibial/fibular junction)
- *Arthritis* (with massive effusion, a "dancing patella" can be palpated)
- *Bursitis* (bursitis prepatellaris and Baker's cyst are most common)
- Pigmented *villonodular synovitis* is a benign neoplasm of the synovium
- Axial alignments (*Genu valgum and Genu varum*) and
- Instability of the joint as the foundation for *OA*
- *Arthropathies* (hemophilia, gout, hemochromatosis, neuropathic)
- Aseptic osteonecrosis (*Ahlbäck's* disease)

4.10.3
Instability of the Joint

- Patellofemoral instability, a clinical diagnose, the cause is traumatic episode
- Cruciate ligament rupture and lesions
- Collateral ligament rupture and lesions

Knee pain may be referred from ipsilateral hip disease or may be due to a neurologic condition resulting from degenerative arthritis of the lumbosacral spine, lumbar disc herniation, or spinal stenosis.[12]

4.11
Hips

Clinical:

- Pain in the pelvic girdle, outer side of the upper leg, anterior thigh pain, radiating as far as the knee, and is associated with hip clicking
- Restricted mobility, mostly on adduction, as far as joint block
- Tenderness around the hips (*Trochantor major*, *M. glutaeus medius*, *among others*)
- Unremarkable imaging (conventional X-ray) is consistent with *Periarthritis coxae* and *Trochanteric bursitis*, respectively

4.11.1
(Sub) Acute Pain

(Also at rest) and joint block

- Pelvis and hip fracture
- *Aseptic osteonecrosis* (see Fig. 121)
- *Acute arthritis*
- Ligament ruptures
- *Ischialgias*
- *Tumor* (metastatic or osteosarcoma)

4.11.2
Chronic Recurrent Pain

- *Inflammatory OA*, with or without *osteitis* (Fig. 97), dysplasia
- *Arthritis*, *rheumatic* (*RA*; *SpA*, Fig. 119), and *infectious* (gonorrhea, TB)

- *Enthesiopathies, periarthropathies* with calcification, trigger points
- *Bursitis* (trochanteric, iliopsoas, ischial/ischiogluteal)
- *Meralgia paresthetica* (compression of the *lateral femoral cutaneous nerve*)
- *Aseptic osteonecrosis*
- "Severe" *low back pain* syndrome
- Difference in leg length

4.12
Spinal Column

(See Chap. 2)

In one third of the population, the *back pain* associated with *STD* has no (radio) morphological correlate; primarily it involves muscle strain (*tendomyosis*) or tension associated with *fibromyalgia. Poor posture*, which is to be regarded both as a consequence of and cause for degenerative *spine* diseases, as well as asymmetrical and inappropriate overexertion and possibly weakened back muscles, is important.

The *most common causes* of *back pain* with a (radio) morphological correlate are presented in the following figure and corresponding CS:

- *SpA* (Figs. 60, 117, 119, 120)
- *Spondylodiscitis* (Figs. 48ab)
- *Sacroiliitis* (Figs. 44–46, 124)
- *Osteochondrosis, spondylosis* (Figs. 116, 118, 123)

Sintering of the vertebral bodies with fractures and paraplegia (Figs. 125–127).

Paraneoplastic Syndromes (PNS) in Rheumatology

5

5.1
Case Description

CS 73 Definite Wegener's granulomatosis (WG) as a mask for colon cancer, male patient 40 years

- The case involves a 40-year-old man, whose symptoms seemed harmless to begin with. In 2 months, there was a subacute development of the following symptoms:
  - Sinusitis with nasal bleeding
  - Arthritis
  - Outbreaks of sweating, and weight loss
  - Highly positive cANCA with high-grade CRP and ESR
  - Morphology: chronic granulomatous ENT changes were ascertained.
  - Such constellations would certainly match *WG*. Cortisone with CYC (approx. 42 g in total) was administered. The patient was very quickly relieved of his symptoms, and remained so for 7 months.
  - Then, the *other side* of the disease emerged, making an almost fulminant appearance:
  - The same, nonspecific symptoms and unusually severe signs of inflammation
  - Check-up revealed:
  - Sonogram – liver metastases
  - Liver biopsy – adenocarcinoma
  - Coloscopy – colon carcinoma

The patient died 14 months later.

Subsequently, it is neither *WG* nor *colon carcinoma*, but rather, *in terms of rheumatology*, the *neoplasias* and *tumors associated with rheumatic conditions*, respectively.

In such associations, as in our case, there are basically three possible explanations:

1. That it could be a *tumorous disease with two sides*, whereby the vasculitis is a *paraneoplasia*
2. That there are *two independent diseases*
3. Or, even, that the neoplasia was *induced by CYC*

E. Benenson, *Rheumatology*, Symptoms and Syndromes
DOI: 10.1007/978-1-84996-462-3_5, © Springer-Verlag London Limited 2011

Therefore, it is essential to answer the most important questions in the tumor–rheumatism constellation – *disease-specific, coincidental, or treatment-related?*

In our case, the *primary* disease is without question *colon carcinoma*, which presented over the course of a few months with definite cANCA-positive *WG*. *This side* of the underlying disease is to be regarded as a *unique, remote effect of the tumor* or as a type of *paraneoplasia* in colon carcinoma, which incidentally has not been described *to date*. However, it cannot be ruled out that high-dose CYC influences the fulminant course of this disease.

5.2
An Overall Picture of PNS (Definition, Classification, Morphology, and Incidence)

There are four aspects to be seen with the manifestation of *rheumatic neoplasia* (using examples from our patient population):

1. *Symptoms at a distance to the tumor*, namely true *paraneoplasia* (see definition)
2. *Rheumatic manifestations* with *neoplasias* and chemotherapies:
   - *Mono-arthritis* (e.g., Fig. 54) and *synovioma, vasculitis*-type symptoms with tumors (CS 73), *lymphomas* (KS 56), *leukemia*
   - *General symptoms* with fever in *lymphoma* (CS 59)
   - *Parotid* enlargement in *Sjögren's* syndrome and *MALT lymphoma* (CS 56)
   - *Hypertrophic pulmonary osteoarthropathy* (polyarthritis, clubbing of the fingers (e.g., Fig. 88) and periostitis), associated *with lung malignancies* or *abscess*
   - *Arthropathy* (e.g., gout and amyloid in *myeloma, leukemias, lymphomas, Jaccoud*-like *in carcinoma of the lung*)
   - *Chemotherapy* and *comedication* (interferon-α, growth factors)
3. *Tumor-like symptoms* in rheumatological diseases:
   - Fluoride *monoarthritis/dactylitis* (Fig. 41, CS 14), this patient with early *RA* (incidentally RF and anti-CCP-Ab highly positive) was operated on suspicion of a tumor prior to study these parameters
   - *Masses* with *RA* in the lungs (Figs. 36a, 38, and 39), bones (Fig. 36b), soft tissues (Figs. 122a,b)
   - *Unclear lymphadenopathy* in *Sjögren's* syndrome (CS 49) or *Still's* disease (CS 66)
   - *Dramatic weight loss* with swallowing difficulties in *CREST* syndrome (CS 58)
   - *Fever, CRP, GGT,* and *LDH elevations of unknown etiology* in adult-onset *Still's* disease (CS 62)
   - *Masses* with *WG* (histologically confirmed) in the sinuses (Fig. 86) or *retrobulbar granuloma* (Fig. 96) or in the uterus (rarely an isolated attack with *WG*) or in the lungs with *caverns* (Figs. 75 and 112)
   - *Massive bihilar lymphadenopathy* with pulmonary masses, in our case with *histiocytosis X* (Fig. 79), gives rise initially to the question of a tumor
4. A *creeping transmutation* of the rheumatic diseases into a *lymphoproliferative disease*, e.g., with *RA* or *Sjögren's* syndrome (CS 56).

Definition: *PNS* involves *symptoms* associated with neoplasia but *distanced from the tumor* which have *nothing to do with either tumor growth or metastasis*. *PNS* occurs in 2–15% of cancer patients.

Pathophysiology: *Biologically active substances* produced by a tumor and antibodies, arising from a cross-reaction, against various antigens (autoantigens, oncoproteins, RNP, and Sm associated with rheumatic diseases), mediate a number of metabolic, hormonal, and immunological changes, which may long have existed during the preclinical phase of a tumor as *predictors*, manifested as *PNS*. The consequence is also a polymorphic, clinical pattern of *PNS*.

Classification: Differentiation is made between various forms of *PNS*, describing them as the *tumor masks*:

- *Internal*
  - *Rheumatological* [1, 4, 9, 11, 17][1]
  - Endocrinological
  - Gastroenterological
  - Nephrological
  - Pulmonological
  - Cardiological [8]
  - Hematological [14]
- Dermatological
- Neurological

Morphology: Rheumatological *paraneoplasias* can in principle appear in *all structures of the connective tissue*, and *all rheumatic syndromes and even categorized diseases* could be induced by neoplasias. Among them are *obligatory* (more seldom) and *informal* (most often) *paraneoplasias*. Two examples of the almost obligatory skin changes in gastric and bronchial carcinoma, respectively: *Acanthosis nigricans maligna* and *Erythema gyratum*.

On the *incidence* of rheumatologic *neoplasias*: old data from the USA give a figure of 1.7%. Our data (observation period of about 4 years, with 2,500 patients) revealed that a tumor or rheumatic *PNS* in fact occurred in 1% of our rheumatic patients.

5.3
Clinical Aspects

5.3.1
The Most Common Admission Diagnoses with PNS

Rheumatological investigation ensues in the following clinical constellations, primarily in patients over the age of 45 years:

- Weight loss, swallowing difficulties, anemia, lymphadenopathy
- *Fever of unknown origin*, resistance to antibiotic therapy

---

[1]Literature references for this chapter only [1–19] can be found at the end of the chapter.

- *ESR* and *CRP elevations* of unknown origin
- Investigation of existing cases of *arthritis, CTD*, and *vasculitis*

In *PNS* patients examined more closely, the clinical constellations were unusual. There was always an inconsistency between the criteria and the pattern of involvement. It is of particular significance that the rheumatic diseases exist up to some years *prior* to the tumors (in one of our cases a female patient with confirmed PM/DM died after 5 years from undetected *breast* cancer).

In everyday rheumatology practice we see a number of rheumatic diseases and their relationships with different tumors (see below), or the *primary* tumors (see Fig. 54), which wear a rheumatological mask.

5.3.2
Vasculitis or *Vasculopathies* and *PNS*

The most common rheumatological forms of **PNS** have been measured by incidence and odds ratio relative risk (*OR*) *as compared with* the entire population [2, 5, 8].

- *Vasculitis* (0.5% identified as being associated with neoplasia), predominantly:
  - *Vasculitis, leukocytoclastic* (Fig. 56, CS 20, 56). Broad consideration should be given thereby to the following:
    - Infections
    - *Allergy*, drug-induced
    - *Tumors* (most common form with tumors, above all with hematological neoplasias)
    - *Systemic vasculitis* (Chap. 13.8)
  - *Wegener's granulomatosis* [18]:
    - Often associated with tumors (*OR* = 1.79), especially with renal carcinoma (*OR*=8.73)
    - Neoplasias that in isolated cases may induce such a disease
    - Every patient should undergo tumor screening
  - *Polymyalgia rheumatica* (tumor screening required by diagnostic criteria)
  - Other forms of *vasculitis* may, in our experience, predominate as *paraneoplasias (Takayasu's arteritis, polyarteritis nodosa)*
- *Vasculopathies (cancer-associated vascular disorders)* are to be regarded as *cardiological paraneoplasias*:
  - *Thrombotic conditions (Trousseau's* syndrome)
    - *Thrombophlebitis superficialis*, migratory
    - Unclear thromboembolisms, arterial and venous (paradoxical embolisms)
    - Deep-vein thrombosis
    - Arterial thrombosis
    - Nonbacterial endocarditis with possible embolization
    - Cardiac thrombosis

- *Atherosclerotic changes*
  - Rapidly progressive ischemic cardiomyopathy
  - Peripheral arterial occlusive disease (as in Fig. 14)
- *Raynaud's* syndrome, *digital gangrene*, as in Fig. 47 (presented in case report)
- Selective incidence of vasculopathies with difference carcinomas, e.g., in *colon carcinoma*, a coronary event occurs up to *40 times* more often than with other tumors [8]
- *Erythromelalgia* (Chap. 9.2.10) can be associated with myeloproliferative disorders and *polycythemia rubra vera*

5.3.3
Connective Tissue Diseases and PNS

- *Dermatomyositis* (as in Fig. 94)
  - Solid tumors $OR = 2.4/3.4$ (men/women)
  - For ovarian carcinoma $OR = 16.7$
  - Tumor as a cause of death 40% [4, 9, 15]
- *Polymyositis*
  - Solid tumors $OR = 1.7/1.8$ (men/women)
  - For bronchial carcinoma in men $OR = 5.6$
  - Tumor as a cause of death 14%
- *SSc* and *SLE*-type syndrome
- *Sjögren's* syndrome (*non-Hodgkin's lymphoma OR* = 10 to 44; CS 56)

The long-term risk of *lymphoma* is estimated to be on the order of 5%.

The presence of low serum C4 or palpable purpura in a patient with Sjögren's may *predict* the development of *lymphoma* [12].

5.3.4
Arthritis/Soft-Tissue Rheumatism and PNS

Neoplasias are known to be associated with *asymmetrical* and *atypical arthritis*, (usually the knee or other large joint), hence tumor screening should always be considered. Such an association has been investigated thoroughly in *RA*, as follows [7, 11]:

- *Solid tumors* are *less common* than in the normal population
- The incidence of *colorectal carcinoma* is *only half as high* (possibly due to the regular intake of NSAIDs)
- A higher risk of
  - *Leukemia* (*OR*=2.5–1.4)
  - *Lymphoma* (*OR*= 19–23.0)
  - *Multiple myeloma* (*OR*= 1.8–5.0)
  appears to be *obligatory and disease-specific*.
- The incidence of lymphoproliferative diseases increases with the duration and activity of *RA*
- Neoplasias, and primarily the incidence of *NHL*, are especially high in *Felty's* syndrome (CS 68).

The associations with *RA* and hematological tumors differ from those with solid tumors that attack the connective tissue from a distance. In principle, neoplasias in *RA* are not paraneoplasias in the context of the definition above. The lymphomas in *RA*, and more often in *Sjögren's* syndrome, emerge from the combination of these two diseases (B-cell activation, Epstein–Barr virus infection) and should be regarded as a consequence of the transmutation of *polyclonal* B-cell activation typical to such autoimmune diseases into *monoclonal* B-cell activation. They are typical for *lymphoma* and in the case of *RA* require investigation.

- *Soft-tissue rheumatism*
- The association of tumors with the following syndromes has been presented in case reports
  - *Fibrosing palmar fasciitis* in ovarian carcinoma (with the impressive description *"unusual and memorable"* [19]), reflecting all the clinical difficulties of *paraneoplasias*
  - *Panniculitis, Erythema nodosum* (Fig. 109), *Lupus profundus* (as in Fig. 27), associated in our case with myeloproliferative disease, which was not further differentiated
  - *Hypertrophic osteoarthropathy* (Fig. 88, → Chap. 3.11.4) associated with bronchial carcinoma
  - *Myasthenia* syndrome (*Lambert–Eaton*) → Chap. 9.6.2

5.3.5
Treatment-Related (Secondary) Neoplasias

Treatment-related neoplasias develop almost inevitably from strong immunosuppression, which could result more or less in decreased host defense and a well-controlled immune response (monitoring). Such a discussion was initiated by the transplant community [10].

First, it emerged that *each transplant patient* on average developed *more than one tumor* in subsequent years, the cause for which was the strong immunosuppression regimen. Hence the incidence of *lymphoma* is much higher in *liver recipients* (17.3%) than in *kidney recipients* (0.16%). Successfully transplanted kidney patients, however, died *significantly more often* from *tumors* (10-year *neoplasia* mortality rate 26%) than dialysis patients (1%), for instance. Such effects were also proven in *RA* and other *arthrologic* disorders under:

- CYC and other alkylating agents [3]
  - All tumors *OR*=4.1 (vs. *RA* control) and 3.7 (vs. total population)
  - *Leukemia* and *lymphoma OR*= 14.6
- Methotrexate showed, in contrast to in vitro, neither mutagenicity nor carcinogenicity (e.g., compared with CYC). Most clinical studies confirm these findings [6].
- Azathioprine demonstrated a minimal mutagenic risk (in one female patient/CS 30/ such an effect is not ruled out; the other/CS 34/, who received a dose that was twice as high/120 g/for 6 years, is tumor-free at present).

- Ciclosporin – no genetic risk
- TNF blockers revealed no increased incidence of tumors in *RA* and *AS* (follow-up for ~10 years) to date, but recently some cases of
  - Hepatosplenal *T-cell NHL* (Chap. 10.10.3) have been reported in young men
  - Increased risk of solid tumors in patients with *WG* who had histories of exposure to *CYC* and were exposed to etanercept [16]
  - Increased early lung cancers in patients with severe COLD treated with infliximab [13]
- *Combined therapy* for tumors

5.3.6
Criteria for the Suspected Diagnosis of PNS

When is the development of a *neoplasm to be suspected* or *when* must such an idea be prioritized during diagnosis in rheumatology patients?

- Age>45 years
- Unclear *B symptoms* (fever, weight loss, anemia)
- Unclear *CRP and ESR elevations*
- *Trousseau's* syndrome or, e.g., in unstable *coronary artery disease*
- *Atypical symptoms* or constellations (as an example):
  - Acute development of florid *arthritis* associated with bone pain or
  - Suspected *polymyalgia rheumatica* in a patient under 50 or
  - Abnormal lab findings, e.g., *monoclonal gammapathy* or *cryoglobulins* (Fig. 132) or
  - Poor, *inadequate response to cortisone* or other therapy (e.g., vasodilation)
- Known, disease-specific association such as *lymphoma* in *RA* or *Sjögren's* syndrome
- Conditions in which *PNS* could emerge from the *remote effect* of solid tumors – the most common being *DM/PM, vasculitis, hypertrophic osteoarthropathy, fasciitis*, among others
- *High-dose immunosuppression* and conditions in which *secondary neoplasias* are suspected, particularly when administering medications associated with a high risk of malignancy, e.g., *CYC* or *polychemotherapy* of tumors

5.4
Special Significance of PNS in Rheumatology

- *Neoplasias* are associated *relatively frequently* and *not just by chance* (in 1–1.7% of patients) *with rheumatological diseases*. They could be classic, histologically confirmed diseases or rheumatic syndromes that *mimic* the already existing neoplasm.
- Rheumatological diseases or conditions far *precede tumor diagnosis* and metastasis (up to 5 years); hence consideration must always be given to *hidden* neoplasm.

- Diagnosis during this phase should focus on a *curative* influence with respect to the entire prognosis.

- Any persistent *B symptoms* and deterioration in *general health* in elderly patients should be viewed as the non-metastatic symptoms of a tumor.

- Such symptoms should be investigated as part of an *integrated diagnostic program* Chap. 13.3) *for the purposes of tumor screening*, as well as *in all*, even local, rheumatological problems.

- *Tumor screening* is necessary in particular in patients
  (a) With neoplasia-associated diseases (*primary neoplasias*) and
  (b) On strong immunosuppression and/or chemotherapy (*secondary neoplasias*)

References

1. Abu-Shakra M, Buskila D, Ehrenfeld M, et al. Cancer and autoimmunity: autoimmune and rheumatic features in patients with malignancies. *Ann Rheum Dis*. 2001;60:433–441.
2. Bachmeyer C, Wetterwald E, Aractingi S. Cutaneous vasculitis in the course of haematological malignancies. *Dermatology*. 2005;210:8–14.
3. Baltus JAM. The occurence of malignancies in patients with rheumatoid arthritis treated with cyclohosphamide: a controlled retrospective follow-up. *Ann Rheum Dis*. 1983;42:368–373.
4. Bernatsky S, Ramsey-Goldman R, Clarke A. Malignancy and autoimmunity. *Curr Opin Rheumatol*. 2006;18:129–134.
5. Blanco R, Martínez-Taboada VM, Rodríguez-Valverde V, García-Fuentes M. Cutaneous vasculitis in children and adults. Associated diseases and etiologic factors in 303 patients. *Medicine (Baltimore)*. 1998;77:403–418.
6. Bleyer WA. Methotrexate induced Lymphoma? *Editorial J Rheumatol*. 1998;25:404–407.
7. Hemminki K, Li X, Sundquist K, Sundquist J. Cancer risk in hospitalized rheumatoid arthritis patients. *Rheumatology (Oxford)*. 2008;47:698–701.
8. Naschitz JE, Yeshurun D, Eldar S, Lev LM. Diagnosis of cancer-associated vascular disorders. *Cancer*. 1996;77:1759–1767.
9. Naschitz JE, Rosner I. Musculoskeletal syndromes associated with malignancy (excluding hypertrophic osteoarthropathy). *Curr Opin Rheumatol*. 2008;20:100–105.
10. Penn I. Incidence and treatment of neoplasia after transplantation. *J Heart Lung Transplant*. 1993;12:328–336.
11. Racanelli V, Prete M, Minoia C, et al. Rheumatic disorders as paraneoplastic syndromes. *Autoimmun Rev*. 2008;7:352–358.
12. Ramos-Casals M, Daniels TE, Fox RI et al. Sjögren's syndrome. In: Stone JH, ed. A Clinician's Pearls and Mythos in Rheumatology. Springer Science+Business Media B.V., Dordrecht Heidelberg London New York. 2009:107–130
13. Rennard SI, Fogarty C, Kelsen S, et al. The safety and efficacy of infliximab in moderate to severe chronic obstructive pulmonary disease. *Am J Respir Crit Care Med*. 2007;175:926–934.
14. Reuss-Borst MA. Rheumatic and hemato-/oncological disorders [Article in German]. *Z Rheumatol*. 2005;64:3–11.
15. Sigurgeirsson B, Lindelöf B, Edhag O, Allander E. Risk of cancer in patients with dermatomyositis or polymyositis. A population-based study. *N Engl J Med*. 1992;326:363–367.

16. Stone JH, Holbrook JT, Marriott MA, et al. for the Wegener's Granulomatosis Etanercept Trial Research Group. Solid malignancies among patients in the Wegener's Granulomatosis Etanercept Trial. Arthritis Rheum 2006;54:1608–1618.
17. Stummvoll GH, Graninger WB. Paraneoplastic rheumatism–musculoskeletal diseases as a first sign of hidden neoplasms [Article in German]. *Acta Medica Austriaca*. 2002;29:36–40.
18. Tatsis E, Reinhold-Keller E, Steindorf K, et al. Wegener's granulomatosis associated with renal cell carcinoma. *Arthritis Rheum*. 1999;42:751–756.
19. Wright GD, Doherty M. Unusual and memorable. Paraneoplastic palmar fasciitis and arthritis syndrome. *Ann Rheum Dis*. 1997;56:626.

Algorithms in Articular and Musculoskeletal Disorders: Integrated Diagnostic Screening Program

6

Staged Diagnostics

To correctly determine the clinical pattern of arthrology and achieve the objective of your work – a confirmed diagnosis – in an optimal way, the diagnostic process is structured and presented here using practical, consecutive steps.

Step 1: Lead symptoms to be documented in as much detail as possible.

Diagnosis should begin, as far as possible, with the full documentation of the rheumatologic patient's *individual symptoms*. Specific questions or *reasons for rheumatological investigations* are useful, and may be addressed on the first visit as follows:

1. *Pain and/or functional disorders* of the joints, back, muscles, or other structures of the musculoskeletal system, posing the question of exclusion of a *primary rheumatic disease* (Chaps. 1.1, 2.1.5, 9.6.1)
2. *Diffuse pain symptoms* (pain everywhere) with no clinical or laboratory evidence of inflammation, fatigue of unknown etiology. So there is the diagnosis already (Chap. 3.5)
3. *B symptoms* of unknown etiology (Chaps. 1.6–1.7, 8)
4. *Organ* (e.g. polyserositis, lungs) or *system* (lymphadenopathy, hemolytic anemia, thrombocytopenia) *involvement* (Chap. 1.6)
5. *Dryness* syndrome, *hair loss* (Chaps. 1.6, 10.7.1, 9.1.6)
6. *Skin eruptions, nodules* on the fingers and joints of unknown etiology (Chaps. 3.1, 9.4.2)
7. *CRP and/or ESR* elevations of unknown etiology (Chaps. 1.6, 8.4)
8. Acute *arthritis* or *dactylitis* of the first toe, increased uric acid (Chap. 1.5.3)
9. Proof of *Borrelia* antibodies (Chap. 11.3.4) with or without evidence of tick bites
10. Proof of *rheumatoid factors, ANA, HLA-B27* (Chaps. 6.7, 11.1)
11. Creatine phosphokinase (*CK*) elevation in the serum (Chap. 9.6.4)
12. Suspected presence of an *immune defect* (Chap. 13.3)
13. *Referrals* from other colleagues (neurologists, ophthalmologists, ENT specialists, dermatologists, gynecologists) for further causal examination of the existing rheumatic symptoms, if applicable (Chaps. 1.6, 11).

Step 2: Which structures are diseased? The question of *morphological diagnosis*.

An attempt is made, when recording the history and undertaking clinical examination as well as during later imaging procedures, to define the *venue* of the connective tissue disease. The simple question of where the problems lie – in the *joints, muscles, spine,* or

E. Benenson, *Rheumatology*, Symptoms and Syndromes   **77**
DOI: 10.1007/978-1-84996-462-3_6, © Springer-Verlag London Limited 2011

extra-articular structures – is not always easy to answer and should be approached systematically. It is the first and most important approach when formulating a diagnosis. The *morphological considerations* can lead us specifically to the relevant syndromes and disease subgroups. These associations are illustrated in Rheumatology

Tree 1 (*RCS*, Chap. 1.3).

Diseased connective tissue structures must be documented by their clinical findings as follows:

1. *Pain, with or without swelling*, in the entire joint surface during movement or rest is suggestive of *diseased joints*.
2. *Run-in pain* in the large joints and fingers suggests involvement of *the joint* (degenerative form) or *tendon sheaths* (inflammatory form).
3. *Back pain*, depending on the pattern of involvement and imaging results, could – rheumatologically – suggest, at the same time, involvement of the *spine, bone* (*osteoporosis, neoplasias*), and *STR* (*tendomyosis*), as well as other internal problems.
4. *Local pain* (e.g., hand, elbow, shoulder, and heel) with *painful movement deficits* when maintaining passive mobility may suggest the involvement of *periarticular* and *soft-tissue* structures, respectively.
5. Muscular pain (*myalgia*) and weakness (*myasthenia*), as well as *elevated CK*, are associated to a considerable degree with *muscular involvement*.
6. *Widespread pain* (everywhere) in the extremities and back is consistent, in elderly and younger patients pretreated with cortisone, with bone involvement (*osteoporosis, Sudeck's* syndrome), or even – mostly in younger women – with *fibromyalgia*.

To *objectify* the morphological diagnosis, *imaging procedures* (*RCS*, Chap. 1.1.1) must be performed, namely

1. *Conventional X-rays of the*
   - Musculoskeletal system, focusing on specific changes in
     - *RA* (Figs. 9ab, 51, 59)
     - *AS* and other forms of *SpA* (Figs. 22, 60, 117, 119, 120)
     - *Gout* arthritis (Fig. 130b)
     - *Sacroiliitis* (Figs. 44, 124)
     - *CTD* (non-erosive arthritis, Fig.72)
     - *OA* (Figs. 8, 97, 128b)
     - *Osteochondrosis* (Figs. 116, 123)
     - *Calcaneal spur* (Fig. 108)
     - *Bony* masses (Fig. 37)
     - *Osteoporosis* (monitoring postoperatively, Fig. 125)
   - Thorax focusing on pulmonary involvement in rheumatic and other diseases
     - *Rheumatoid nodules, tumors,* or *TB* (Figs. 36a, 38)
     - *Wegener's* disease (Fig. 75)
     - *Sarcoidosis* (Fig. 91).
2. *Two-phase bone scan* (Figs. 49b, 64, 65b) enables the pattern of involvement to be objectified and solves the question: Is there any increased uptake of the radionuclide in

the musculoskeletal system or other organs, and if so, are there any changes that are inflammatory, noninflammatory, or suggestive of a tumor?

3. *Ultrasound* of the joints and tendon sheaths provides clarification of whether there are any effusions or ruptures in the respective structures.
4. *CT* is used to diagnose diseases and conditions involving the *musculoskeletal system* (as an example):
   - *Destructive bone involvement* (Figs. 23, 34)
   - *Osteoporosis* with fractures (Figs. 125–127)
   - *Hyperostotic spondylosis* (Fig. 118)
   - Investigation of unclear forms of *monoarthritis* (Fig. 54), in this case a suspected *bone tumor*, indeed a *stress fracture*.

   CT of the thorax should be used to investigate suspicious tumorous masses, e.g., *rheumatoid nodules* in the lungs (Figs. 36a, 38, 39).
5. *MRI* is reported to be the best imaging method for differentiating *local soft-tissue and bone marrow changes* and for monitoring therapy for:
   - *Chondromalacia*, sport-related (Fig. 26)
   - *Active sacroiliitis* (Fig. 46)
   - *Spondylodiscitis* (Figs. 48a, b)
   - *Plantar fasciitis* (Figs. 98, 99)
   - *Tendinitis, osteitis, enthesitis* (Figs. 102, 103)
   - *Shoulder pain* syndrome (Figs. 106, 107)
   - *Aseptic necrosis* of the acetabulum (Fig. 121)
   - *Tumor*-like mass or massive *rheumatoid nodules* in the lower arm (Figs. 122a, b) or leg (Fig. 36b).

The ultimate outcome of the morphological considerations should define, in as much detail as possible, the *venue* of the disease – namely whether the *joints and/or spine* are involved, or specifically the *periarticular structures* or *STR*? Thereby, it is important to resolve issues which must be approached with different methods as regards extra-articular changes Rheumatology Tree 1 and 2 (*RCS*, Chaps. 1.3–1.4). The explanations on diagnosing syndromes with such structural involvement are given in this book, Chaps. 1–3.

Step 3: Are there inflammatory or noninflammatory changes in the musculoskeletal system? The question of *pathophysiological diagnosis*.

Identification of diseased structures and the *morphological substrate* of the disease appear to be the *most important* and at the same time *most difficult* task for the clinician. The next question is: What are the changes that have taken place?

The common clinical symptoms affecting the joints (*arthralgia, swelling, movement deficits*) may certainly complicate matters when differentiating between *arthritis* and *osteoarthritis (OA)*.

Inflammatory involvement of the *joints, muscles, and soft-tissue structures* is characterized in principle by the following symptoms, which by nature can in any case vary (by intensity, majority, and scope) and be entirely *isolated* or *combined* (Chaps. 1–3):

- *Pressure pain* (with the exception of *tender points* in *fibromyalgia* and the points beyond *panalgesia* syndrome)
- *Swelling*, with or without warmth
- *Effusions* in the joints, bursae, tendon sheaths
- *Painful nodules* (*Heberden's, Bouchard's, rheumatoid nodules, gout*)
- *Limitations to active movement*
- *Morning stiffness* (a diagnostic criterion and activity parameter in *RA* and *AS*)
- *Pain at rest* (a sign of the activity of *inflammatory back and joint pain*).

Noninflammatory involvement of such structures is linked to further clinical factors:

- *Pain without* the above mentioned symptoms
- *Load-dependent pain* (typical of *OA* and *spondylosis*)
- Limitations to *passive movement* (*contractures, ankyloses, (sub)luxations*)

Such a question – *inflammatory and/or noninflammatory changes* – is particularly important to *back pain* (Chap. 2) due to the delayed diagnosis of *AS* (average 6.4–10 years). The only explanation for an *inflammatory pain pattern* not being detected thereby, despite clear guidelines having been standardized in all textbooks (see too Chap. 2.1). The described feature of *back pain* should at least bring to mind the concept of *SpA*. The concomitant clinical (*arthritis, enthesitis, scleritis*) and laboratory (*CRP, ESR*) inflammatory parameters could certainly confirm such a suspicion.

An *inflammatory pattern of involvement* in the extra-articular structures (Chap. 1.6) presents in the form of similar, local clinical symptoms as with joint involvement (see above), but could at the same time be triggered by *mechanical* and *inflammatory* processes.

Consideration must be given thereby to:

- Suspected *enthesitis, tendinitis, osteitis* should be confirmed by a *bone scan* and *MRI*
- The presence of a systemic inflammatory disease (*RA, SpA, CTD, vasculitis*), particularly if system or organ involvement has been confirmed (Chaps. 10, 13.5), is indicative of an inflammatory process.
- The *spine* changes are associated with certain diseases and their activities. In *primary vasculitis*, it is essential to define where and which types of morphological processes are actually taking place or have occurred (Chap. 13.4).

On account of such symptoms and considerations it should as a whole be clear whether *the inflammatory or noninflammatory* changes are taking place in the musculoskeletal system (Rheumatology Tree 1 and 2, see **RCS**, Chaps. 1.3–1.4).

Step 4: Pattern of articular, spinal and soft-tissue symptoms. The question of *nosological entity*.

So we have already managed to differentiate between the four subgroups of rheumatic diseases (*arthritis, OA, arthropathy, STR*), which have common morphological and pathophysiological characteristics. The overall impression is very helpful, but not sufficient. Further nosological differentiations are made between the joint diseases on the basis that *every rheumatic disease* has its own *specific pattern of involvement*, which must be identified as the next essential diagnostic step. The features defined in the *diagnostic criteria* for *joint and spine* symptoms are reflected in the *pattern of involvement*, and vice versa.

In understanding the pattern of involvement, the distinctions between *arthralgia, arthritis, OA*, and *arthropathy*, above all, must be determined at the given time. Accordingly, the question arises as to *which of these four forms of articular change is primarily involved?*

With the exception of *arthralgia*, which must be investigated in a particular way (Chap. 1.1), the remaining syndromes are suggestive of the disease subgroups (Rheumatology Tree 1, see *RCS*, Chap. 1.3). The distinctions between the diseases in which the syndrome of *arthritis* or *OA* predominates are particularly varied and of much importance. To establish the *arthrological pattern of involvement* ultimately entails finding a solution to the following questions:

1. *Which of these syndromes* occurred *with the onset* of the joint problems?
2. Is it *monoarthritis*, i.e., affecting just one joint, or *oligoarthritis* (affecting up to three joints) or *polyarthritis* (more than three joints)? Each of these forms of arthritis is associated to a large extent with certain diseases.
3. Are the *large and/or small* joints involved?
4. Is the pattern *symmetrical or asymmetrical*?
5. Are there any *erosive* or *non-erosive* changes (on X-ray)?
6. What about *development*: chronic progressive, (sub)acute or episodic?
7. Are the *joint problems* associated *with back pain*?
8. Is there any *morning stiffness* in the joints and spine, and *how long* does it last?

These articular features are the shortcut to one entity.

Spine involvement (Chap. 2) is classified in a similar way to joint diseases (Chap. 1). The diagnosis of *SpA* is often used as a generic term for undifferentiated, inflammatory *spinal* diseases, which, in accordance with the criteria, should be defined as one of seven *seronegative forms of SpA*, namely:

- *AS*
- *PsA*
- *ReA*
- *Enteropathic arthritis* or *arthropathy*
- *HLA-B27*-positive *oligoarthritis*
- *SAPHO* syndrome
- *Undifferentiated SpA*, if a case cannot be assigned to any of the given diagnoses.

Degenerative spine changes or diseases are derived from the respective scans (Chap. 2.3) as

- *Spondylosis, spondylarthrosis, osteochondrosis*
- *Discopathy*
- *Spondylosis hyperostotica*
- *Spinal canal stenosis* syndrome.

STR is divided into two subgroups (Chap. 3). *Inflammatory STR* is ascertained clinically and by MRI (see above) as associated with *SpA* (*enthesitis, tendinitis,* and *osteitis*) or *RA* (*tendinitis*) or as *one entity* (*panniculitis, fasciitis*). Local, *mechanically induced* periarticular changes also have inflammatory aspects (confirmed clinically and by MRI), but are often regarded as *noninflammatory STR*, i.e., *tendinosis, panniculosis, enthesiopathy.*

Step 5: Association with infections, tumors, other diseases. Questions: *causal diagnosis, idiopathic or secondary, condition or disease.*

Causal diagnosis defines the clinical pattern and the course, the treatment strategy, and its prognosis in the case of more than 200 rheumatic diseases and conditions.

The background to this is:

- The *connective tissue* and *immune system* originally derived from the mesenchyme are almost always involved and often affected by every action and disease
- True rheumatic diseases are idiopathic (*primary* rheumatic diseases), others causally related to or associated with infections and non-rheumatic diseases (*secondary* rheumatic disorders)
- *Tumors*, as a cause of rheumatological symptoms or true rheumatic diseases, are estimated in 1% of our patients. Hence consideration must inevitably always be given, in every case and particularly in patients over 45 years, to *tumor* screening (Chap. 5)
- In principle, *each connective tissue symptom* must be afforded broad and precise consideration and follow-up in terms of *all potential non-rheumatic diseases and causes*, as well as be ruled out
- *Idiopathic diseases are at present restricted to just a few forms* (*RA, Still's, JIA, AS, PsA, CTD, primary vasculitis, polymyalgia rheumatica, fibromyalgia*); hence precisely these diseases should be incorporated in the diagnostic circle if, in the case of connective tissue or system/organ symptoms, the other causes have been ruled out.

Step 6: System-organ involvement. Question: *systemic or local problems.*

The *background* to this step is:

- Rheumatic syndromes and diseases are to be regarded as *local and/or systemic problems*; *screening* for *systemic* involvement must commence *as early on as possible*
- Diagnosis of a *local rheumatic disease or condition* should ensue *after exclusion* of *systemic involvement.* If the localized problems predominate, e.g., *spondylodiscitis* (Fig. 48), *sarcoidosis* (Figs. 83, 90), *osteolysis* (Fig. 34), *panniculitis* (Fig. 27), or *fasciitis* (Fig. 95), an *extensive check-up* is desirable, with consideration not least of *tumors, infections,* and as yet undetected organ involvement
- *Mono symptoms,* e.g., *monoarthritis,* some cutaneous (*vasculitis, psoriasis vulgaris*) and/or subcutaneous (*Erythema nodosum*) changes, should initially be regarded *by no means as a localized problem*
- The existing *B symptoms* (*fever, lymphadenopathy, CRP elevation, anemia*) of unknown etiology are mostly consistent with *systemic involvement*

- If *CTD* or *vasculitis* is suspected, *all systems and organs* also comprising connective tissue structures (vessels, interstitium, immune system) should be examined thoroughly and specifically (in just the same way as an extensive tumor screening program)
- In the case of *inflammatory joint, spinal*, and *STR* symptoms, concomitant diseases or conditions must be actively investigated. The most common among these are
  - *Psoriasis* (Figs. 84ab, 110, 111, 129b), in relatives such evidence has equal importance, in ~5% it may entail no skin changes (CS 8, Fig. 23; CS 23, Figs. 68, 88)
  - Chronic *Yersinia* (CS 40, Fig. 109) or *streptococcal* infection with *Erythema nodosum*
  - Inflammatory intestinal *(arthropathy)* and ocular (*ReA, SpA*, Fig. 57) diseases
  - Genitourinary symptoms and diseases (in *ReA, SpA, gonorrhea, Behçet's* disease)
  - *Reddening* of the skin (*Erythema migrans* from tick bites confirms the diagnosis of borreliosis) or joint, almost certainly a *gout* (Fig. 13) or *septic arthritis*
  - *Ulcerations* of the mucous membranes (Fig. 76, *Behçet's, CTD*, CS 64, *vasculitis*)
- *Every extra-articular symptom* must be investigated for *systemic involvement* or associated diseases.

Step 7: Investigation of inflammatory, immunological, and serological activity.

Together with system-organ manifestation, such parameters define *nosological categorization, present activity* of the diseases, the *treatment strategy*, and approaches to *monitoring*.

Inflammatory activity is a generic term covering clinical and laboratory data that can provide information on the extent as well as the floridity and scope of the inflammatory components.

- *Clinical* parameters:
  - Deterioration in *general health*, particularly with a view to fatigue and mobility
  - Duration and intensity of *morning stiffness*
  - *Exudative arthritis* or *tenosynovitis*
  - *Number of swollen joints* and extent of *spine* involvement
  - *Intensity of tenderness* in the joints
  - *Painful restriction to movement* (according to intensity and extent of block)
  - *Cortisone dependency* (according to daily dose)
- *Laboratory* parameters (Chap. 8.4):
  - *CRP* (rapid indicator of inflammation of varying etiologies, *cave* tumors)
  - *ESR* (delayed indicator of inflammation, remaining more or less stable in CTD, other conditions)
  - *Acute-phase proteins* (fibrinogen, ferritin, alpha-1 and -2 fractions in serum electrophoresis)
- *Synovial fluid* parameters correlate with the *activity* of *arthritis* and should be categorized as
  - *Noninflammatory* (*transudate*, typical of inflammatory *OA*)
  - *Inflammatory* (*exudate*, typical of nonbacterial *arthritis*) and
  - *Bacterial* (exudate is typical of *septic arthritis*).

At the same time, *synovial analysis* is important to nosological diagnosis, involving the following tests:

- *Leukocyte count* (between 3,000 and 50,000/µL) is an indication of *exudate* (compared to transudate)
- Neutrophil count (25–75%; 90–95% is highly suspicious of *RA, crystal* and *septic arthritis*)
- *Rhagocytes* (immune complex-based, spherical neutrophils) are highly specific in *RA*
- *Hemorrhagia* (*arthropathy* in *hemophilia* Chap. 1.5.4 or rarely *tumors* of the synovia)
- *CRP* (on the issue of differentiation between exudates/arthritis and transudates/osteoarthritis)
- *Crystals* (uric acid in *gout* and others in *pseudogout* → Chap. 1.5.3)
- *Viscosity* (increased with *exudates*, normal with *transudates*, found most commonly in *inflammatory OA*)
- *Immunological diagnostics* (rheumatoid factors, possibly DNA-Ab)
- *Microbiological diagnostics (pathogen detection in bacterial forms of arthritis: PCR for Chlamydia trachomatis, borreliosis,* and *septic forms of arthritis* in noncultivable bacteria)
- *Synovial biopsy* demonstrates the extent of mononuclear infiltration or inflammation, confirming the diagnosis of *RA*
- *Imaging procedure*
  - *Polyarthritic involvement* in *bone scan*
  - *Massive articular effusions* (*arthrosonography, MRI*)
  - Extensive *osteitis* on *MRI* (in *arthritis, SpA,* and *inflammatory OA*)
- *Combined clinical parameters*
  - *DAS 28, BASDAI* (score 3.5 and above)

Immunological and serological activities are associated with *active inflammatory joint disease* (Chap. 11.1.1):

- *Rheumatoid factors* (RF) are not always correlated to inflammatory activity in *RA,* but more to the severity and extra-articular processes; low-titer RF could be "false positive" (in ~6–25%, depending on age, CS 28, 47, 53)
- *Anti-CCP*-Ab (for early identification, and a prognostic parameter, as CS 14 shows; surgery can thus be avoided; *sensitive to a limited extent in early forms*)
- *ANA* (CS 32, 53) could, in seropositive *RA,* be indicative of other diseases
- *ACE and IL-2r* (in *sarcoidosis,* CS 33 as follow-up and other diseases)
- *Cryoglobulinemia* (CS 20)
- Serological diagnostics revealed *high-grade* antibodies. Antibody detection is to be evaluated only within the context of the clinical findings:
  - *Antistreptolysin O* (*rheumatic fever*); with no clinical findings, it was falsely evaluated (CS 71)
  - *Yersinia (IgA),* pivotal to the diagnosis (CS 37, 40, 60)
  - *Borrelia* (IgM/IgG, possibly in the liquor), ~95% in the serum have no clinical correlate
  - *Chlamydia trachomatis*

- *Pathogen diagnostics* in the form of direct detection by culture or PCR (in *ReA*). Detection of *pathogen antigens* confirms the diagnosis:
  - *Fecal culture (Yersinia, Salmonella)* with symptoms of diarrhea or positive serology
  - *Synovial analysis* (for *Chlamydia trachomatis and Borrelia burgdorferi*)
  - *Urine (morning urine) and vaginal smears (Chlamydia trachomatis)*
- Determination of *HLA-B27* antigen (88–96% association with *AS* or *SpA*) is to be interpreted more as a *genetic predisposition* and never as an *activity parameter*.

Step 8: (Radio) morphological pattern of disease.

Relevant objective parameters represent an obligatory component of diagnostics in *rheumatology* and are of *pivotal importance* in *joint and spine* diseases. It is best to employ the appropriate methods in a *certain sequence*, irrespective of the clinical situation and the specific issues.

Conventional X-ray is indispensable if inflammatory or degenerative *joint and spine* diseases are suspected, particularly to diagnosis and DD, severity and staging, follow-up controls, and defining the surgical consequences. The *hands and forefeet* should be X-rayed as a minimum. *CT and MRI* are further, practically inexhaustable possibilities in terms of morphological imaging diagnostics and are suited for monitoring both progress and effectivity.

The most important *lead symptoms and syndromes* from *morphological imaging*:

8.1 *Arthropathies*

I. *Syndrome* of *exudative* and *proliferative arthritis* (Fig. 22):
   A. *Early signs* of *arthritis*
      1. *Distribution in soft tissue*, arthritic collateral phenomenon as well as
      2. *Demineralization (near the joints)*
   B. Direct signs of *arthritis*
      3. Joint space narrowing, symmetrical, or concentric
      4. Atrophy of the subchondral border lamella
      5. Usures, cystic defects
      6. Osteoblastic proliferations (protuberances) are typical of *PsA*
II. *Syndrome* of *fibrosing–ankylosing, destructive arthritis* (Figs. 9a, 51, 59):
   1. *Erosions*
   2. *Cystoid* osteolysis in the vicinity of the joints
   3. Mutilations (deep-seated substance defects, *"pencil-in-cup"* phenomenon)
   4. Ankyloses
   5. Deviations
   6. Sub/luxations
III. *Syndrome of osteoarthritis* (Figs. 8, 97, 128b):
   1. Osteosclerosis (joint vicinity)
   2. Joint space narrowing, asymmetrical
   3. Osteophytes
   4. Usures
   5. Chondromalacia (Fig. 26, *MRI*)

IV. *Other syndromes*:
1. Osteonecrosis (Fig. 121)
2. Osteolyses (Figs. 23, 34, 36b, 37, 54, 96)
3. Calcifications (Fig. 18)
4. Periostitis

8.2 *Spinal* diseases

I. *Spondylarthritis (SpA)*
1. Erosions (Figs. 45 *CT*, 119, 120 at the *symphysis*)
2. Syndesmophytes (Figs. 60, 117, 124)
3. Joint space narrowing (Figs. 44, 119)
4. Spondylolyses (contour defects in the end plate, as in Fig. 48a, *MRI*)
5. Ankyloses (Figs. 117, 124)
6. Sclerosis (Figs. 116, 117, 119, 124)
7. Capsule-disc-ligament calcifications
8. Plantar fasciitis (Figs. 98, *MRI*; 108, *conventional X-ray*)
The most important conditions of *SpA* are to be identified on the basis of such changes:
* *Sacroiliitis* (Figs. 44 and 124 *conventional X-ray*, 45 *CT*, 46 *MRI*)
* *Spondylitis* (Figs. 60, 117, 124)
* *Spondylodiscitis* (Fig. 48a)
* *Symphysitis* (Figs. 119, 120).
II. *Spondylarthrosis* (Figs. 116, 118, 123, 127, *CT* Thorax)
1. Reduced intervertebral space (*chondrosis*)
2. Increased subchondral sclerosis (*osteochondrosis*)
3. Erosions (*erosive osteochondrosis*)
4. Space narrowing of spine joints (*spondylarthrosis*)
5. Disc changes
6. Formation of marginal spikes or spondylophytes (marginal and hyperostotic)
7. Sondylosclerosis

8.3 *Objectification* of clinical diagnosis

To this aim, the questions already discussed above are addressed:

8.3.1 The question of *differentiation* between (in order of frequency) *STR, degenerative or inflammatory, and tumorous* diseases should first be answered, namely in:

* *Two-phase* (blood pool/Figs. 49b, 65b/and a late phase/Fig. 64/) *bone-joint scan:*
  * *Pathological enhancements* in the musculoskeletal system or other organs mostly do not support organic diseases, though in individual cases they are not ruled out
  * *Pathological enhancements (hot spots)* are suggestive of diseases or conditions
  * *The pattern of involvement* of the *enhancements,* above all the asymmetric involvement in *sacroiliitis,* is the next step and the key to further diagnosis

The low specificity of such a screening method is to be considered, particularly when addressing *arthritis* or *inflammatory OA*; false-positive and false-negative results are not uncommon.

8.3.2 Screening for *disease-specific changes* takes the form of:

- *Conventional X-rays* of the hands and feet, as well as sacroiliac joints and spine, while questioning:
  - *Erosive and other specific changes* in:
    - *RA* (Figs. 9ab, 51, 59), *gout* arthritis (Fig. 130b), *PsA* (Chap. 1.3)
    - *Degenerative joint diseases* (Chap. 1.4; Figs. 8, 97, 128b)
    - *Arthropathies (Paget's*, among others)/Chap. 1.5/
    - *AS (syndesmophytes)* → Chap. 2.2.1; Figs. 60, 117, 119, 120
    - *Sacroiliitis* (Chap. 2.2.3; Figs. 44, 124)
    - *Degenerative spine diseases* (Chap. 2.3; Figs. 116, 123)
    - *Spondylosis hyperostotica*/DISH/(massive spondylophytes → Chap. 2.3.2; Fig. 118 in CT)
    - *Calcaneal spur*/plantar fasciitis/→ Chap. 3.7.2; Fig. 108
    - Complications (bone fracture, *aseptic necrosis* → Chaps. 3.10, 3.11; Fig. 125)
    - *Osteolyses* (CTD, vasculitis, hyperparathyroidism)
  - *Osteoporosis, local or diffuse* (this method is indicative only if at least 30–50% of the bone mass has been lost → Chap. 3.11)
- *DEXA (dual-energy radiographic absorptiometry)* is the safest method for diagnosing *osteoporosis*
- *Arthrosonography* is one of the modern means of dynamic diagnostics, and helps in the detection of
  - Soft-tissue lesions (*periarticular edema, synovial proliferation,* tendon and muscle *ruptures,* scarring)
  - Accumulation of fluid in the *joints and tendon sheaths* (*bursitis, tenosynovitis*)
  - Bone lesions (contour defects, erosions, osteophytes, loose bodies)
  - Calcifications, and
  - Articular punctures (diagnostic and therapeutic)
- *Doppler sonography* in
  - *Pannus and vascularization* diagnosis in MCP and PIP joints with *RA*
  - *Arteriitis temporalis (giant cell arteritis* diagnosis).
- *CT* and *MRI* for fine diagnosis of *articular, STR* and *spine* diseases. *CT* mostly reveals the *scope and nature* of the joint destruction, bone and organ involvement. *MRI*, unlike *CT*, involves no radiation load and is to be regarded as having the best resolution with no overlap as well as being the best dynamic method for differentiating between *local soft-tissue and bone-marrow* involvement, and for diagnosing activity:
  - *Bones (osteolyses)* and *soft-tissue* involvement
    - *CT*
      - *Erosive oligoarthritis* in HLA-B27 positive female patient (Fig. 23)
      - *Osteolysis* of unknown etiology/*"vanishing bone disease"*/(Fig. 34)
      - *DISH* (diffuse idiopathic skeletal hyperostosis) syndrome (Fig. 118)
      - *Sacroiliitis* when staging (Fig. 45)
      - *Bone fractures* in osteoporosis with myelon involvement (Figs. 126, 127a)
      - *Orbital granuloma* in *Wegener's* disease (Fig. 96)

- *MRI:*
  - *Rheumatoid nodules* in the bones (Fig. 36b)
  - *Large rheumatoid nodule* mass in the soft tissue in female *RA* patient (Figs. 122ab)
  - *Sacroiliitis* in activity assessment (Fig. 46)
  - *Spondylodiscitis* in *AS* (Figs. 48ab)
  - *Osteolysis* with *stress fracture* (Fig. 54); DD in primary *bone tumor*
  - *Osteonecrosis* (Fig. 121)
  - *Plantar fasciitis, tenosynovitis, osteitis* (Figs. 98, 102, 106)
- *Organ involvement*:
  - *CT:*
    - *Rheumatoid nodules* in the lungs (Fig. 39)
    - *Pulmonary fibrosis* possibly in *RA* or under MTX therapy, as in Fig. 53 (in *SSc*) or Fig. 85 (in *MCTD*)
  - *MRI:*
    - *CNS* involvement possibly in *RA*, as in Fig. 50 (in *Sjögren's* syndrome)
- *Histology* for diagnosis (Chap. 11.6) of
  - *CTD*
  - Secondary *vasculitis*
  - *Polyneuropathies* (in *RA* and *ReA*) and *sarcoidosis*
  The aim here is not always to obtain a groundbreaking finding, in which clinically apparent changes are identified (Figs. 20, 32).
- *Capillary microscopy* for diagnosis of *secondary vasculitis* and *CTD* (*SSc, MCTD*) or *primary Raynaud's* phenomenon (no pathological findings in comparison to *secondary Raynaud's*).

Negative results in terms of such findings do not rule out these conditions.

8.3.3 The disease activity must be objectified by:

- *Bone scan* (polyarthritic pattern of involvement)
- *MRI* (extensive *osteitis*)
- *Skin-muscle biopsy* (cell-rich lymphoplasmocytic infiltrations)

8.3.4 The *severity of the joint and spine changes*, i.e., erosions, joint space width, ankylosis, cartilage-bone destructions, *compression* syndrome, is ascertained by:

- *Conventional X-ray* of
  - Hands in *RA*, measured by
    - *Lars score and Sharp score, grade 0–5*
  - Cervical spine in *AS* and *RA* (destructions and *atlantoaxial dislocations* in segment C1/C2)
  - Sacroiliac joints in *SpA*
    - *Sacroiliitis* in *SpA* is assessed semiquantitatively, *grade 0–4.*

Other joints are assessed selectively and according to indication, using the same morphological criteria.

- *CT* and *MRI*
  - *Dislocations* of the cervical spine
  - *Slipped discs* and cartilage defects
  - *Spinal canal stenosis*
  - *Tumor diagnostics* and masses in the lungs, liver, aorta, periaorta, and retroperitoneum (*Ormond's* disease)
  - *Spondylodiscitis*
  - *Carpal tunnel* syndrome
  - Proof of *osteonecrosis* (MRI)

8.3.5 *Follow-up* over the course takes the form of:

- *Conventional X-ray* of hands, feet, sacroiliac joints with a view to bone destruction
- *Two-phase bone* and joint scintigram with a view to the skeletal pattern of distribution
- *CT* with a view to existing dislocations, slipped discs, stenosis
- *MRI* with a view to existing *osteitis, osteonecrosis*

8.3.6 *Organ involvement* (lungs, kidneys, etc.) is documented as a standard (Chap. 10)

Step 9: Preliminary diagnosis and consistency with recognized diagnostic criteria.

As a result of structured consideration of the morphological, pathophysiological, nosological, and causal aspects of a disease (Steps 2–6), thereby enabling *differentiation* at every step, the clues to preliminary diagnosis have been obtained.

- With respect to the syndromes, the question should firstly be addressed as to whether a *primary disease* or a *condition* exists
- Further, a *morphological, pathophysiological, and causal diagnosis* should be formulated on the basis of the clinical syndromes
- Subsequently, the diagnosis is objectified and specified more precisely on the basis of imaging, morphological (Step 8), and laboratory (Step 7) procedures. Such considerations facilitate the correct diagnosis or help to ascertain whether diagnostic criteria are lacking
- *Diagnosis is confirmed* by making a *comparison with known diagnostic criteria* of the disease or syndromes.

Step 10: Diagnostic formulation.

Thus we have reached the endpoints in our medical endeavors. The *diagnosis of a disease* must take the following components into account:

1. *Entity*
2. Major *syndromes* representing *the morphological substrate* of the disease
3. Clinical *activity*
4. *Course* of the disease (sub/acute, progressive, stable, remission)
5. *Immunological features*
6. Changes found *morphologically* or confirmed by *imaging*

7. *Complications*
8. *Status following therapy* or *postoperatively* with
9. *Therapeutic complications*
10. *Concomitant diseases*
11. Major rheumatic and non-rheumatic *concomitant syndromes*

When *diagnosing a condition* that entails only a morphological diagnosis, the following must be taken into account:

- *Morphological and pathophysiological characteristics* with *patterns of involvement* (i.e., Steps 2, 3, and 4 of such a screening program need to be defined)
- *Which primary diseases* are possibilities with such a condition (Step 5)?

Such a *diagnostic formulation* and *syndrome-oriented, diagnostic program* are consistent with the coding recommendations for rheumatology[17] and have been presented as examples for arthrological (CS 69, 70) and other diseases (CS 71–72 in *RCS*, Chap. 1.2 and CS 73 in this book, Chap. 5).

This screening program, adapted to *articular* and *musculoskeletal disorders*, has much *in common* but to a certain extent also *differs* from the screening program presented in Chap. 13 for *CTD* and *vasculitis*.

These *similarities* can be found in the *integrated diagnostic screening program* (*RCS*, Chap. 1.1) and are applied *to all clinical disciplines*.

Algorithms in Arthrological and Musculoskeletal Disorders

7.1
From Lead Symptoms to Syndromes

There is no standardized diagnostic pathway. Some colleagues take the *lead symptoms* as the most common starting point when ascertaining a diagnosis, while others place great value on obtaining *specific laboratory measurements and images* or finding the *most common combinations* of symptoms; other experienced colleagues look at the *syndromes*. The selected data are compared against known diagnostic criteria.[1, 9, 10, 26]

Whatever the approach, consideration of *diagnostics as a process* is essential, whereby *selective screening* for a specific laboratory test or imaging method, and *visual diagnosis* or enlightenment are not seen as the ideal objective, since this requires more specialized thought processes. The journey entails *contemplation* of what lies behind these symptoms and patterns, *the morphological, pathophysiological, and etiological conclusions to which they lead*, while considering the body as a whole. Only in such a way can the existing condition, and if possible the disease, be identified. The approach is somewhat more complicated perhaps, but safer for sure.

This diagnostic pathway – *from symptom to disease* – requires experience, and for good reason is often followed by experienced physicians and always by young doctors and students. Priorities are thereby placed on experience, associations, and memory. Experienced colleagues thus are quick to reach the correct diagnosis, as soon as they have briefly, and almost subconsciously, asked themselves the questions, *"Which structures are affected?"* and *"Are there any inflammatory or noninflammatory changes?"*

Students should use their powers of recall and association (they should always have the diagnostic criteria of some diseases to hand), and/or available sources of information. This journey – from symptom to disease – *is to be viewed as a continuation of the information-oriented, descriptive teaching associated with medical work* and at the same time the only opportunity for students to perform their tasks effectively.

Such reasoning has been discussed in several books.[12, 15, 25] The chapters of these books dedicated to arthrology (*back pain* and *joint pain*) list all related diseases, which without doubt is both essential and useful in equal measure to the extensive considerations of internal medicine.

Much in the same way as the extensive XXL checklist "Differential Diagnosis of Internal Medicine",[25] wherein the guideline *"From symptom to diagnosis"* presents a "clear and up-to-date source of information for daily clinical practice."

Despite the justified question of whether such a guideline – from symptom to diagnosis – actually reflects the everyday reasoning in medical practice (certainly not to the full extent), we shall attempt to observe this guideline, limiting ourselves here to arthrological and musculoskeletal problems. We are of the opinion, however, that between *symptoms* and *diseases* we should find the *syndromes* – as the proper morphologically, pathophysiologically, and causally defined elements of diagnosis.

Nevertheless, the individual symptoms, or rather their stable combinations, i.e., syndromes, could be the *driving force* behind the ascertainment of a disease by way of sorting the illnesses that come into question. We have not taken individual symptoms as the starting point for diagnostic consideration, but rather their most common combinations (Table 7.1).

7.2
From Syndromes to Diseases

As soon as the syndromes are linked to the connective tissue structures and their pathophysiology and potential causes investigated, the next step should be taken, namely to define the disease(s) (Table 7.2).

7.3
Therapeutic Algorithms (as an Example in RA)

7.3.1
Common Principles

These algorithms should represent the latest, most important therapeutic strategies in arthrology. The venue, the objectives, and the specialist fields involved, as well as the number of patients, are so extensive and multifarious, that emphasis should first be placed on narrowing the specialization. Patients with inflammatory rheumatic diseases, even those suspected of such, should at least have one consultation with a rheumatologist specialized in internal medicine (the situation at present is such that only *one patient in four is seen by a rheumatologist*). At this point, further difficulties with rheumatology care emerge.

Patients with *degenerative joint* and *spine* diseases should primarily be treated by *orthopedic specialists*.

Patients with *localized problems* (florid arthritis, inflammatory OA, compression and facet syndromes, soft-tissue disorders) within the context of systemic inflammatory and degenerative diseases should be treated by their *family doctors and all specialists* (in orthopedics, rheumatology, nuclear medicine, physiotherapy) with a view to the lead symptoms, whereby local therapy should be deemed an adjunct to optimal systemic treatment (at least for inflammatory rheumatic diseases).

Table 7.1 Diagnostic pathways from leading symptoms to syndromes

	Most common symptoms in stable combinations	Syndrome
1	One or more joints swollen with tenderness and loss of function	Mono-/polyarthritis
2	Deformity, contracture, ankylosis	Outcome of arthritis
3	Morning stiffness	OA, arthritis
4	Pain and stiffness in the back, umbosacral region, in the morning, improving after movement	Spondyloarthritis, sacroiliitis
5	Arthralgia and back pain of "mechanical" nature	OA, spondyloarthrosis
6	Widespread chronic pain (in the joints without swelling, muscles, back) associated with fatigue	Fibromyalgia, panalgesia syndrome
7	Myalgia, tenderness in the muscles, myasthenia	Myositis
8	Arthralgia, tenderness over the joint line, limited activity, but normal passive motion of the affected joints	Periarthropathy
9	Pain and limitation of active motion in one or two fingers, worse upon awakening, thickened, tender volar sheaths on palpation (Fig. 95)	Tendinitis, tenosynovitis
10	Heberden's (Figs. 3, 4), Bouchard's (Figs. 4, 128ab) nodes	OA of the finger joints
11	First carpometacarpal joint painful or swollen	OA base of the thumb
12	Acute monoarthritis with redness, broad swelling of the MTP 1 or quite rare MCP 2 right (Fig. 13)	Acute gout arthritis, Septic arthritis
13	Tophi, periarticular (Fig. 130b), at the helix of the ear	Chronic tophaceous gout

(continued)

Table 7.1 (continued)

	Most common symptoms in stable combinations	Syndrome
14	Rheumatoid nodules (Figs. 3, 35, 104, 129c)	Extra-articular manifestations of RA
15	Sicca features (oral and ocular dryness –xerostomia and xerophthalmia)	Sjögren's syndrome
16	Fever, weight loss, lymphadenopathy, neuropathy, organ involvement	Systematic extra-articular manifestations of joint diseases
17	Erythematous swelling on the auricular part of the ears with sparing of the earlobe (Fig. 29)	Auricular chondritis most likely in a setting of the Relapsing polychondritis
18	Connective tissue findings in neoplasia	Paraneoplastic syndrome
19	Connective tissue findings in neurological, endocrine, hematological, metabolic disorders, sarcoidosis	Arthropathy
20	Clubbing of the fingertips/toes/and convexity of the nail contours (Fig. 88)	Hypertrophic osteoarthropathy (paraneoplastic syndrome, intra-thoracic infections, among others)
21	Dactylitis (Figs. 41, 65ab)	ReA, PsA, SpA, RA, SAPHO syndrome, Lyme borreliosis, gout
22	Numbness and tingling in digits 1–3, loss of sensation in the affected fingers, thenar muscle atrophy	Carpal tunnel syndrome

Table 7.2 Diagnostic pathways from syndromes to disease(s)

	Syndrome	Diseases
1	Morning stiffness in and around the joints lasting at least 1 h, over a period of more than 6 weeks	RA
2	Stable (for more than 6 weeks) arthritis of the PIP, MCP, and MTP (except the end joints) with erosions and joint deformities (Figs. 9ab, 35, 40, 49ab, 58ab, 129a)	RA
3	Arthritis, with neither erosions nor deformities (Figs. 28, 41, 70, 72)	Early RA, CTD, ReA, and other forms of arthritis, vasculitis, paraneoplastic syndromes
4	First MTP joint painful or swollen, unilateral involvement, chronic recurrent tophi, bony erosion by tophi, removed from the joint space (Fig. 130b)	Gout arthritis, pseudogout
5	Asymmetric peripheral (oligo or mono) arthritis, often with predilection for the DIP, PIP, and MCP joints (Fig. 64, Dig. 3 left)	PsA
6	Arthritis of the peripheral large joints, asymmetric and oligoarticular, and axial (spine and sacroiliac joints), non-erosive, possible infection of the gastrointestinal or genitourinary tracts, associated with extra-articular manifestations	ReA
7	Arthritis of the lower extremities and large joints (most affected), asymmetric, low back pain, heel pain (as in Figs. 102, 108)	SpA, AS
8	Neck, back pain (nocturnal, worse with rest, improves with activity and after NSAIDs), accompanied by morning stiffness	SpA, AS
9	Non-stabile, migratory arthritis of the large joints associated with streptococci, virus, and other infections	Rheumatic fever, ReA, Lyme borreliosis, gonococcal, and other infections
10	Run-in pain in peripheral joints, increasing with activity and relieved with rest, brief morning stiffness, disability	OA

(continued)

Table 7.2 (continued)

Syndrome		Diseases
11	Osteoarthritis with synovial inflammation in the form of mono-oligoarthritis (Figs. 4, 81), usually associated with overload (Fig. 25)	OA with synovitis
12	Heberden's (Figs. 3, 4) and Bouchard's (Figs. 4, 128ab) OA (with localized tenderness and bony or soft tissue swelling)	Interphalangeal OA, e.g., with synovitis
13	Extra-articular systemic changes in erosive arthritis (Figs. 35–39, 55, 100, 101ab) or SpA (Fig. 57)	RA, SpA, SLE, chronic gout arthritis
14	Systemic changes in non-erosive arthritis (Figs. 70, 72)	CTD, systemic vasculitis
15	Mechanical low back pain and disability increases with physical activity, with neither inflammatory findings in the blood nor sacroiliitis	Spondylosis, spinal osteoarthritis
16	Pustular keratoderma blemorrhagica (Figs. 110, 111, 129b)	Pustular psoriasis, SpA, ReA, SAPHO syndrome

7.3.2
Therapeutic Concepts

Inflammatory rheumatic diseases (*RA, AS, PsA*) have common strategies:

1. *Objectives*: induction and maintenance of remission or drug-free state, improvement in quality of life
2. *Prerequisite*: certain diagnosis
3. *Principal direction*: immunomodulation, primarily immunosuppression
4. *Points of attack*: activation and dysregulation of the immune system (T cells, B cells, macrophages)
5. *Primary indications*:
   - Early forms with curative approach
   - Unfavorable, also prognostic, variant of the diseases:
     - Polyarticular involvement and high-grade activity
     - Refractory course
     - Increased cortisone requirement
     - System and organ involvement
     - High immunological activity
6. *Principal methods:*
   (A) *Systemic therapy*:
   (I) Chemical immunoactive products
     - Glucocorticosteroids (also as pulse therapy) act as DMARDs in *RA*
     - MTX
     - Azathioprine (also as pulse therapy[3])
     - CYC (also as pulse therapy)
     - Ciclosporin
     - MMF (Cellcept®, Myfortic®)
     - Leflunomide (Arava®)
     - Gold preparations
     - Sulfasalazine
     - CP-690,550, Tasocitinib® (oral antagonist of Janus kinase 3, as part of a phase 3 study, Chap. 12.3)
   (II) Biologics (for *RA, PsA, AS, psoriasis vulgaris, JIA*)
     - TNF-*blockers (first line* for all approved substances) should be given main concomitantly with MTX
       - Enbrel®/*etanercept*, 25 mg×2 or 50 mg weeks, *SC*, possible without MTX up to achieving a response or remission followed, if necessary lay-off of therapy; applies to other biologics
       - Remicade®/*infliximab*, 3 mg/kg – *IV* infusion initially and at in 2, 4, 6 weeks
       - Humira®/*adalimumab*, 40 mg×1 in 2 weeks, *SC*
       - Cimzia®/*certolizumab* pegol, 400 mg initially and at weeks 2 and 4, followed by 200 mg every 4 week, *SC*
       - Simponi®/*golimumab*, 50 mg given once a month, on the same date each month, *SC*

- B-cell *inhibitor* (anti-CD20 and 19)
  - Mabthera®/*rituximab, second line* for *RA*, 500–1,000 mg *IV* first and after second week, then expected remission for a mean of ~14 months
    - Ocrelizumab® (anti-CD 19, as part of a phase 3 study)
- IL-6 *receptor blocker*, RoActemra®/*tocilizumab*, as *first-line* biologic for *RA*, 4–8 mg/kg *IV* infusion × 1 in 4 weeks
- *Inhibitor of costimulation*, fusion protein, Orencia®/*abatacept*, for RA as *first line; IV* dose based on weight: less than 60 kg, 500 mg; 60 to 100 kg, 750 mg; more than 100 kg, 1 g. Subsequent doses at 2 wk, 4 wk, and every 4 wk thereafter.
- *IL-1* receptor antagonist, Kineret®/*anakinra*, 100 mg *SC* every day
- *IL-1* dimeric fusion protein is able to tightly bind IL-1, *rilonacept*
- *IL-1* Ab Ilaris®/*canakinumab*, 2 mg/kg or 150 mg *SC* every 4 months

In *Still's*, *CAPS*, and other *autoinflammatory diseases* (Chap. 8.1), and *gout*, in which IL-1 overproduction plays a key pathogenic role, these last three drugs with peculiar mechanism seem to be effective

(III) Allogenic bone marrow transplantation (in the refractory patients on the above mentioned therapies with *SLE, SSs, relapsing polychondritis, sarcoidosis*)

(B) *Local therapy* (independent meaning in *mono-/oligoarthritis* and *sacroiliitis*), mostly combined with systemic therapy:
- Radiosynoviorthesis (RSO)
- Cortisone preparations
  - Lederlon® and others (triamcinolone acetate), mostly intra-articular
  - Lipotalon® (dexamethasone palmitate) in inflammatory *STR*
- Early synovectomy

7. *Rational principles*:
- Earliest possible ascertainment of indication
- On induction: highest tolerable doses of basic preparations during the specified period (e.g., MTX 20–25 mg/week, preferably *SC*, up to 3–6 months, aiming for combination thereafter)
- Combination of basic preparations (e.g., MTX + Arava® possible in *RA*)
- On maintenance therapy: lowest possible doses of DMARDs and cortisone ("safe" doses of Decortin® up to 7.5 mg per day)
- Biologics are to be more widely used, promptly and in line with the indication
- Use of approved biologics for early disease (e.g., Enbrel® for *RA*)
- Combination of systemic and local therapy
- Combination with NSAIDs (in *SpA* and *RA*)
- Strict adherence to contraindications
- Active prevention and therapy for real and potential side effects

8. *Selection* and application of *adequate immunological parameters* for prescription and monitoring of therapy (e.g., CRP, RF, B-cell count)
9. *Careful follow-up* with clinical and imaging (X-ray, arthrosonography, MRI) procedures

7.3.3
Algorithms of Individualized Therapy

Such presumed guidelines for therapy can be deduced from the *special variants*, the *activity*, and the expected *severity* of the diseases. As a result, they are linked to specific diseases but also tend to have *more similarities* (*than differences*) in inflammatory rheumatic diseases on account of the shared venue and similar profile of the autoimmunological and inflammatory activities (Table 7.3).

TNFα antagonists and other *biologics* (refer also to Chap. 12.3) are an enormous therapeutic enhancement in the treatment of severe forms of inflammatory rheumatic diseases. Current recommendations of the Food and Drug Administration, USA, on *TNF blockers* can be found on the website www.hhs.gov.

7.4
Prognostic Algorithms

Within arthrology, the prognostic factors are first defined with a view to the major inflammatory joint and spine diseases. At the same time they signify the severity of the diseases.

- *Rheumatoid arthritis*:
  - Polyarthritic symmetrical involvement at an early stage
  - Early erosions
  - Extra-articular manifestations have their own prognostic criteria
  - High RF, anti-CCP-Ab, high-titer in particular
  - Autoimmune phenomena (ANA, dsDNA-Ab, cryoglobulins)
  - Rheumatoid nodules
  - Initially elevated CRP and ESR values
  - Poor functionality at 1 year
  - Poor response to steroids (daily requirement for Decortin® 10 mg or more)
  - Advanced age (*late onset)*
  - Smokers
  - Poor compliance and socially disadvantaged

Table 7.3 Rheumatoid arthritis (special forms and variants depending on the course)

Variants		Special forms of therapy
1	Uncertain diagnosis, persistent monoarthritis or oligoarthritis, mild favorable course, single erosions	NSAIDs Hydroxychloroquine (200–400 mg/day) If necessary MTX
2	"Classic form" (~85%), typical distribution of arthritis (symmetric small/spares DIP/and large joints, moderate activity, positive rheumatoid factor and anti-CCP antibody, deteriorating course, radiographic progression, demand for cortisone, incompatibility of some DMARDs (CS 1, 13; Figs. 35, 40, 42, 43, 80, 104, 129c)	Glucocorticoids (prednisone < 10 mg/day) MTX 15–25 mg/week SC, then PO combined with hydroxychloroquine or sulfasalazine (1–3 g/day) Arava® 100 mg about 3 days, then 20 mg/day, or, if needed, combined with MTX (10–15 mg/week) Intra-muscular gold (Tauredon® 50 mg/week) Intra-articular therapy (triamsinolone acetonide 20–40 mg) Radiosynoviorthesis(/90) yttrium-citrate/ Biological DMARDs (see below)
3	Mono-/oligoarthritis, moderate/minimal activity (Figs. 28, 41, 58–59, 65)	MTX 10–15 mg/week, SC or PO or Arava® 20 mg/day Prednisone 20–0 mg/day for 2 weeks Intra-articular therapy (see above) NSAIDs (in any form of RA)
4	Mono-/ologoarthritis, florid, highly active with redness and swelling of the periarticular structures (Fig. 13)	Acute gout arthritis or pseudegout

5	Permanent high activity, rapid course, severe bone destruction (Figs. 49, 129c)	Intra-venous pulses of methylprednisolone (e.g., 250–500 mg about 3–5 days) and then low-dose glucocorticoids (e.g., 20–10 mg/day) MTX 25–30 mg/week SC + folic acid Leflunomide 20 mg/day (if needed, in combination with MTX) Intra-articular therapy (see above) Biological DMARDs (see below)
6	RA with systemic features (extra-articular manifestations), vasculitis, organ disorders, polyneuropathy, rheumatoid nodules, also in lungs, bone (Figs. 35–39, 55, 100, 101ab, 112ab)	Intravenous pulses of glucocorticoids *e.g., methylprednisolone 250–500 mg IV about 3–5 days or *Dexamethasone 8 mg PO for 5–7 days CYC: *Pulse therapy 500–800 mg/m^2 IV monthly about 6 months, then, e.g., consolidation therapy *2 mg/kg/day PO (with normal kidney function) Maintenance therapy: *Prednisone 30–20–10 mg/day PO or *Dexamethasone 3–0.5 mg/day Try to switch to: *MTX and/or leflunomide *Biological (e.g., actemra, rituximab)
7	Felty's syndrome (CS 68)	Glucocorticoids: *Prednisone 40–30 mg, e.g., 10 mg/day or *Pulse therapy (see above), if needed MMF (CellCept® 2 g/day) *Rituximab (label of use)

(continued)

Table 7.3 (continued)

Variants		Special forms of therapy
8	Still disease (CS 66), Adult-onset Still's disease (CS 62, Fig. 131)	Glucocorticoids: *Prednisone 40–30–10 mg/day PO or *Dexamethasone 4–2–0.5 mg/day PO MTX 15–25 mg/weeks SC + folic acid Anakinra 100 mg/day SC Canakinumab (IL-1-Ab) SC Leflunomide (own experience) Tocilizumab (label of use) IV
9	Late-onset RA or combined with OA (CS 32)	Glucocorticoids: *Prednisone 30–10–5 mg/day MTX 10–15 mg/week, SC or PO or Leflunomide 20 mg/day (with MTX, if need) Intra-articular therapy (see above)
10	RA with secondary Sjögren's syndrome (CS 32)	RA (see above) and Sicca syndrome therapy: *Substitutive and oral muscarinic agents *Systemic/glucocorticoids and immunosuppressive agents/for systemic features
11	RA in remission (a) Spontaneous (without medication) (b) Appeared during maintenance therapy	(a) No DMARDs, if necessary NSAIDs (b) First attempt to reduce or remove glucocorticoids, then the DMARDs. NSAIDs or intra-articular therapy (see above)

12 RA with comorbidity, mostly glucocorticoid-induced:

(a) Diabetes mellitus (CS 70)
(b) Osteoporosis
*Clinically significant (CS 46)

(a) Therapy of diabetes mellitus II
(b) Biphosphonates:
*Risedronate (Actonel®) 35 mg/week
*Alendronate (Fosamax®) 70 mg/week
*Ibandronate (Boniva® 150 mg orally once monthly or 2 mg IV every 3 months)
*Zoledronic acid (Aclasta® 5 mg IV every 3 months)

*Silent (supplementing osteoporosis therapy)

Calcium 500/1,000 mg + Vitamin D 500/1,000 mg (adequate daily dose)

Gastrointestinal toxicity
(c) Peptic ulceration of
*Ventriculi/duodeni/colon
*Gastritis, Helicobacter pylori positive

(c) Gastroenterologic investigation and therapy:
*Proton pump inhibitors
*Coadministration of misoprostol
*Amoxicillin 2,000 mg/day – 7 days
*Metronidazol 800 mg/day – 7 days

(d) Gastrointestinal hemorrhage or perforation, or suspected
(e) Clinically significant complications from
*DMARDs

(d) Emergency gastroenterologic investigation
(e) Initial discontinuation
*A second attempt is possible with MTX and leflunomide, also with smaller doses of MTX and prophylactically; combination with folic acid (5–10 mg next day) advisable

*NSAIDs (traditional)

*Coxibs (Arcoxia® 90 mg/day) or
*Painkillers (analgesics)

- *Ankylosing spondylitis*
  - Acute course
  - All sections of the spine affected
  - Rapid ossification of spine and hip joints
  - Spondylodiscitis
  - Initial functional disorders unrelated to an episode
  - Elevated CRP
  - Extra-articular manifestations
  - Poor response to NSAIDs
- *Psoriatic arthritis*
  - Polyarthritic involvement with erosions at early stages, mutilations, and *SpA*
  - High-grade clinical (skin, joints, spine) and inflammatory (CRP) activity
  - Progressive course
  - Systemic organ involvement (eyes, heart, aorta, liver, kidneys)
  - Cortisone required at doses of 10 mg or more daily

Connective Tissue Disease (CTD) and Vasculitis Systemic Diseases in Rheumatology

These large groups of diseases belong to the other half of rheumatology and, with the exception of the relatively rare cases involving orthopedic and surgical complications, are dealt with by specialists in internal medicine and rheumatologists. Here there is a distinction to arthrology, where the majority of patients are treated by orthopedic specialists. The two halves of rheumatology should be given logical consideration, from *one* perspective, on account of their many similarities – as far as establishing the diagnosis (structured syndrome diagnosis and reasoning) is concerned.

Below, the elements of connective tissue disease (CTD) and *vasculitis* are presented, i.e. applied knowledge of the nature, clinical and pathophysiological features of such syndromes. The syndromes shared with arthrology can be found in Chaps. 1, 3, and 4. The routine documentation of the many, often unique symptoms, which nonetheless reflect the *similarities and distinctions* of these diseases, is of much importance to the diagnosis, estimation of the severity, and prognosis of individual diseases of either category and remains a challenge, even to the experienced physician. Preliminary diagnostics should be undertaken by non-rheumatology colleagues, but confirmation of the diagnosis and therapy for such patients – a clear distinction to issues of arthrology which can in many cases be solved through primary care – should ensue after at least consulting a specialist.

Such diseases are extremely variable and inhomogeneous, just as in arthrology. Their *similarities* were initially noted due to their unique *morphology* (fibrinoid degeneration as well as connective tissue and vascular involvement) and the excellent work by Klemperer et al. (1942),[16] who introduced the generic term *"diffuse collagen disease."* Somewhat later, the similarities or *"overlaps"* in the *clinical findings* (undifferentiated connective tissue syndromes, organ involvement, immunological deviations) and *pathophysiology* (immunological activities) became evident; hence the diagnosis of *CTD* (Klemperer P, *Concept of Connective Tissue Diseases*, Circulation1962; 25:869) was for a long time *inevitable*. Due to our lack of knowledge at the time this was a stopgap with respect to differentiating between the pertinent diseases in the event that an entity could not be correctly defined. Today, the term *diffuse collagen disease* may not be used as a diagnosis (if so, then as a suspected diagnosis) since we have become familiar with the clinical and immunological distinctions between the diseases of this subgroup – in the same way as the ultimate diagnosis of *rheumatism* or *vasculitis*.

A *nosological entity* should always be sought as the diagnosis. In practice, the necessary *distinctions* between the various forms of such diseases can only be achieved by careful clinical analysis of the existing syndromes. Using such elements, and applying morphologically or pathophysiologically structured reasoning, it is relatively easy to establish the *nosological entity* vital to therapy and prognosis, even if it is the first encounter with such systemic diseases.

Lead Symptoms and Syndromes in Systemic Diseases

These lead symptoms and syndromes tend to emphasize the *similarity* of such diseases more than their *disease specificity*. The general symptoms and organ manifestations are associated to a very large extent with the activity of the diseases and their sequelae, and differ more in their severity and incidence than in their quality. *Nosological diagnosis is found* less in the screening of relatively rare specific symptoms, and more in the *typical constellations of syndromes* of each disease which represent the morphological, pathophysiological, and immunological features of an entity. Below, these syndromes along with the disease-specific constellations and symptoms are presented in a systematic manner, structured morphologically.

These syndromes reflect the present situation regarding the development of a systemic disease. Over the course, the same syndromes could appear in an entirely different form or combination, leaving the initially documented history of the disease unidentifiable (CS 24). With such a disease, the composition of the *mega syndromes* (Rheumatology Tree 2, see *RCS*, Chap. 1.4), namely the *general connective tissue/organ* syndromes, and more or less specific *(auto) immunological phenomena*, as presented below, remains stable.

To sharpen the clinical senses to syndrome diagnosis and its relative value when assessing disease activity, a score (maximum *63*) is given using the example of *vasculitis* for system/organ involvement which is of particular clinical relevance – as foreseen by the *Birmingham Vasculitis Activity Score (BVAS)*.[19] In a similar way, such a score can be calculated for *SLE* using the *Systemic Lupus Erythematosus Disease Activity Index (SLEDAI)*.[5] They produce scores for the major individual symptoms and syndromes.

By documenting these major syndromes, *damage* arising from previous activity can also be estimated, i.e., by quantitative measurement along the same principles, by means of the *Systemic Lupus International Collaborating Clinics/American College of Rheumatology Damage Index for SLE (SLICC/ACR)*[6] and *Vasculitis Damage Index (VDI)*.[11] The clinical significance of such activity and damage indices is discussed (Chap. 13.8).

Deterioration in general health (B symptoms) or *severe illness* are the most important *expressions* and *similarities* amongst all systemic diseases, suggesting generalization, activity, and rapid progression or complications, and could also be localized forms of *CTD* (e.g., *eosinophilic fasciitis*) or *vasculitis (Panarteritis nodosa)*.

Sub/acute onset of disease with *B symptoms* are typical of all *prognostically unfavorable forms* of *CTD* and *vasculitis*, but also of *Polymyalgia rheumatica* and *giant cell arteritis*. If B symptoms are unclear, consideration is also to be given to non-rheumatic symptoms (*lymphoma*, CS 59, other *tumors, infections, familial Mediterranean fever (FMF), lethal midline granuloma, Ormond's* disease, among others, cf. → Chap. 13, Step 3).

8.1
Fever of Unknown Origin

Fever of unknown origin (FUO) is of pivotal clinical importance.

Definition: repeated fever above 38°C for more than 3 months, the cause of which could not be found.

Most commonly:

- Infections (approx. 50%), most to have responds to antibiotics
- Tumors (approx. 30–35%), to respond neither to antibiotics nor to steroid
- *CTD/vasculitis* (approx. 10–15%), most to have responds to steroids
- and rare entities:
- Periodic fever and autoinflammatory syndromes or diseases
- Granulomatous disease (sacoidosis, Crohn's disease, Erythema nodosum)
- Metabolic and endocrine disease (e.g., Fabry's disease, hyperthyroidism)
- Psychogenic fever (factitious, in a patient with FUO was found the multiple abscesses under the skin and *B. coli* in the pus)
- Undiagnosed (resolved and recurrent)

---

[1]*BVAS (Birmingham Vasculitis Activity Score)*[19] still demonstrates (Chaps. 9 and 10) the importance of the individual systems-/organs in the assessment of vasculitis activity (Chap. 13, Step 8).

E. Benenson, *Rheumatology*, Symptoms and Syndromes
DOI: 10.1007/978-1-84996-462-3_8, © Springer-Verlag London Limited 2011

"*Periodic fever* syndromes" and inflammation can have a genetic origin with an early onset in childhood or beyond the age of 20 years and belong at present to *hereditary auto-inflammatory syndromes* or *diseases*. These conditions are defined as recurrent attacks of generalized inflammation for which neither infections nor systemic causes can be identified. Included in this spectrum is adult-onset *Still's* disease, *Schnitzler* syndrome, *familial Mediterranean fever* (*FMF*), *TNF-receptor-associated disease*, and others (see below).

They are characterized by periodic or recurrent episodes of *systemic inflammation* causing *fever*, accompanied by rash, serositis, lymphadenopathy, arthritis, and other clinical *CTD* und *vasculitis*-like manifestations in barrier tissues (synovial tissue, serous membranes, and the skin). The other large group of autoinflammatory diseases belongs to the *cryopyrin*-associated periodic syndromes/*CAPS*/(*familial cold autoinflammatory* and *Muckle–Wells* syndrome). These are characterized by chronic or recurrent systemic inflammation associated with various clinical presentations, including urticaria-like rash, arthritis, amyloidosis, and sensorineural deafness. In the pathophysiology of the *autoinflammatory syndromes* or *diseases* the increased IL-1β production (one speaks to *IL-1 mediated diseases*) and TNF-α signaling probably plays an important part that has opened up new therapeutic avenues (Chap. 12.3).

In our cases, such a *fever* symptom is predominant in the event of *Takayasu's arteritis* (CS 25, Figs. 74 and 77ab), *Yersinia-induced arthritis* (CS 40, 60), *Still's* disease (CS 62, 66, Fig. 131) and *lymphoma* (CS 59), and *Fabry's* disease (noninflammatory lysosomal storage disease!).

Clinical features of this syndrome in *CTD* and *vasculitis*:

- Most often signifying generalization, an attack or a complication
- Could also be isolated fever (up to 39°C), often for months
- Fever easy to tolerate with *CTD* (e.g., *SLE*) and relatively difficult to tolerate (due to association with other B symptoms) with *vasculitis*
- No sensitivity to antibiotics
- Could have septic aspects: nocturnal sweating (e.g., in *Still's* disease, *SLE*) with secondary infections can always be expected
- *Periodic fever* syndrome associated with
- *Still's* disease, adult-onset (CS 62, Fig. 131) and juvenile (CS 66)
- Recurrent attacks of the same type with *fever* (up to 40°C, lasting between 6 and 12 h to 3–7 days) and abdominal pain (*peritonial irritation* → Chaps. 10.4–10.5), monoarthritis and spontaneous remission, should give rise to the concept of *familial Mediterranean fever*
- Chronic *urticaria* and monoclonale *IgM-gammapathy* and other systemic features is characterized by *Schnitzler* syndrome
- Elevated levels of *polyclonal immunoglobulin D* as well as lymphadenopathy, abdominal pain, and diarrhea
- In *children* with cyclical episodes of fever, consideration should also be given to *cyclic neutropenia* (recurrent attacks of fever at 21-day intervals) and *PFAPA* syndrome (*p*eriodic *f*ever, *a*denitis, *p*haryngitis, *a*phthous stomatitis) and *macrophage activation* syndrome (Chap. 10.10.5)

- Response to *cortisone* (dose-dependent effect) is indicative of *cortisone-dependent disease* or a condition entailing a broad spectrum of differential diagnostics (Chap. 13, Steps *2–3*); response to *colchicine* could suggest *gout arthritis, pseudogout* or *familial Mediterranean fever*
- Response to *aspirin*. Here, we have the *aspirin test* when questioning whether a fever is inflammatory or noninflammatory (e.g., central fever or psychosomatic) in nature

Fever, as a concomitant symptom in *CTD*, seldom exceeds the temperature of 39°C (consideration should be given to an attack), and as a rule is indicative of a *subfebrile nature*. In the event of fever of unknown etiology, *Still's* disease (CS 62, 66, visual diagnostic in Fig. 131), *Takayasu's arteritis* (CS 25) and even *mononucleosis, superinfections* (respiratory-urinary tracts) and sepsis, as well as inflammatory *lipodystrophy* and *panniculits* with fat necrosis should be considered.

8.2 Weight Loss

Weight loss (>10% or >1–2 kg in the previous month) of unknown etiology or *cachexia* (Figs. 10–11), as an initial or early lead symptom, is an expression of severe metabolic disorders. Such rapid development could apply in all forms of *CTD, vasculitis* and *Still's* disease. In our cases such lead symptoms existed with *ANCA-positive vasculitis* (CS 48) due to *intestinal ischemia* or involvement of the small intestine, or with *Takayasu's arteritis* (CS 25), or *SSc* (CS 19), or *CREST* syndrome (CS 58) due to esophageal motility dysfunction.

8.3
Headache

Headache with or without *dizziness*, new or sudden onset and mostly severe, persistent, and resistant to therapy (analgesia), could be migraine; when excluding the most common neurological causes (brain hemorrhage, dural sinus thrombosis, infection, malignancy, etc.), these could be the *lead symptoms* in:

- *Giant cell arteritis* (a diagnostic criterion); often associated with *Polymyalgia rheumatica*
- *CNS* Vasculitis, in primary *antiphospholipid* syndrome (CS 6), *Sjögren's* syndrome (CS 18), *Churg–Strauss* syndrome (CS 72)
- *"Lupus* headaches" is a part of the *SLE* (listed on the SLEDAI)
- *Still's* disease (CS 66)
- *Retrobulbar granuloma* (Fig. 96)
- *Cervical arthritis* and *spine* involvement (CS 63)
- *Relapsing polychondritis* (Fig. 29)

- *Arterial hypertension* (in all forms of *vasculitis* with renal involvement)
- *Reversible cerebral vasoconstriction* syndrome (a "thunderclap" headache is associated with a variety of conditions, including pregnancy, head trauma, exercise, exposure to nasal congestants, and cannabis)

8.4
CRP and ESR Elevations

CRP and ESR elevations of unknown etiology are typical of *CTD* and *vasculitis*, but clinically should be differentiated:

- *Uniform* elevation in *ESR* and *CRP* is typical in *vasculitis*, some forms of *CTD* (e.g., *SLE* with serositis and arthritis), *tumors*; in one male *RA* patient with minimal activity, such a constellation was suggestive of *Polymyalgia rheumatica* (CS 52)
- *Elevated ESR* (disproportionately higher than *CRP*): in *giant cell arteritis, Polymyalgia rheumatica* (over the age of 50 years); *Takayasu's arteritis* (may exceed 100 mm/h), *SLE, antiphospholipid* syndrome (mostly in young women); a rising ESR indicates often the return of some disease
- *Normal ESR* is more useful in excluding almost all these diseases but does not eliminate it altogether
- *Elevated CRP* (disproportionately higher than ESR): *infection, sepsis, Still's,* other *autoinflammatory disease, Yersinia ReA, Sudeck's*
- *Elevated CRP* tends not to be typical in *CTD* (as opposed to elevated *ESR*), possibly indicating *superinfection* or another *complication*, and should be discriminatory in the differential diagnosis of *CTD*, e.g., with *Still's* and other *autoinflammatory* diseases or *vasculitis* or *obesity*
- *Elevated CRP* could enable the cause to be defined more easily if *procalcitonin* is measured at the same time

The increase in procalcitonin is not characteristic of *CTD, vasculitis,* and other inflammatory rheumatic diseases (CS 62, 64), and is very typical of systemic, bacterial and fungal infections, or sepsis (excepting *gout, aspergillosis*). Our patient, a 65-year-old male, had a *fever up to 39*°C for 6 months, and at the same time a *CRP* level of 237 mg/dL (×*47*), *procalcitonin* – normal (0.5 µg/L). In the diagnosis of *Still's* disease, the *prompt response to cortisone* was the deciding factor after ruling out other diseases (Chap. 13, Step 3).

8.5
Fatigue, Exhaustion, Drop in Performance

So-called *CTD fatigue* (in severe cases with functional impairment) also applies to *RA* and systemic *vasculitis*, and accompanies these diseases for years, even after successful treatment. Such nonspecific problems have a broad differential diagnostic spectrum, including *endocrinological, neurological, and psychosomatic* conditions, and sarcoidosis and should be investigated repeatedly, particularly in the event of deterioration.

Most often, the ability to distinguish in the case of serious fatigue between *CTD* and *fibromyalgia* or *chronic fatigue* syndrome (*CFS*) is questioned. It is not always easy to start with on account of other common syndromes, namely, mild fever/37.5–38.6°C/, new onset of headache, unstable *arthralgia*, neuropsychiatric symptoms, *myalgia* and considerable *myasthenia* (until bound to a wheelchair), palpable *lymph nodes*. Despite extensive morphological and pathophysiological investigations (Chaps. 9, 10, and 14), such noninflammatory conditions are not always easy to determine, e.g., in a 45-year-old female (CS 59): 14 years after treatment for *lymphoma*, the original general symptoms intensified, leading to diffuse pain, subfebrility, unstable CRP elevations, and a drop in performance.

The question – relapse, new inflammatory or noninflammatory rheumatic disease – could only be answered over the course and perhaps not conclusively.

Involvement of Connective Tissue Structures

9

The identification of such involvement, together with organ involvement (Chap. 10), is to be interpreted as the indication of an inflammatory rheumatic disease or condition. The combined element of these two mega syndromes is vascular involvement, which should be perceived as *primary* in *vasculitis* or *secondary* in connective tissue disease (*CTD*) and *vasculitis* as well as many other diseases and conditions (infections, tumors, drug toxicity, metabolic, such as *Fabry's* disease). The key to primary forms of *vasculitis* can be found in the morphological categorization of such vascular involvement (Chaps. 9.2.1 and 9.2.2). With secondary forms of *vasculitis*, every vessel (group) could be affected, in principle, thereby defining the myriad of vascular and organ symptoms listed below.

The nature and extent of such general syndromes, of system-/organ involvement and immunological phenomena (Chap. 11), convey the variety and uniqueness of the clinical pattern as well as the severity and prognosis of these diseases. These syndromes, which are listed below, are ultimately a reflection of clinical and morphological changes, characterized partly or solely by the *present activity* and/or by the *irreversible damage* caused. All new or recent symptoms, as well as their deterioration or improvement from, for example, cortisone therapy, are to be evaluated more as signs of activity (Chap. 13, Step 8). Such a dilemma, and the interaction between activity and possibly several forms of damage, could be explained only by thorough clinical testing of the syndromes given below, during the course of the disease. Identification of the primary changes is the major difficulty in the clinical diagnosis of *CTD* and *vasculitis*.

9.1
Skin and Mucosa[1]

(*BVAS*=maximum of six out of 63 points).

These most varied of symptoms, in the case of *CTD* and *vasculitis*, are inseparably intertwined with *vascular changes* (immune complex-associated or other forms of *vasculitis*) and *microcirculation disorders*, and most often appear with the following syndromes. Only a few of these have a certain degree of disease specificity and are therefore included

---

[1]For his useful hints and suggestions during our conversations and discussions, I thank Dr. Ingo Haase (Clinic for Dermatology at the University of Cologne).

in the diagnostic criteria. Not all the changes described below should be interpreted as *vasculitis*. The significant six points on the *BVAs*. represent the lesions (*infarcts, ulcer,* and *gangrene*) associated specifically with tissue damage, as well as *purpura* and *other forms of cutaneous vasculitis*[19]. These syndromes are mostly nonspecific and are indicative of the primarily morphological (connective tissue, vessels, and their size) and pathophysiological (noninflammatory, inflammatory, sclerotic, thrombotic) changes. The skin is the preferred target organ for *CTD* as well as *primary and secondary vasculitis*.

9.1.1
Erythema and Exanthem

Erythema and exanthem is always a sign of inflammatory changes (*dermatitis*), mostly of the *small vessels*. New or renewed onset of such changes is a *sign of activity*. Predominant localizations and nature of cutaneous efflorescences:

- *Bridge of the nose and both cheeks*
  - *"Butterfly rash"* (described in every textbook) is a specific diagnostic criterion of systemic Lupus erythematosus (*SLE*) and has two forms: irregular, diffuse reddening of the skin (*vasculitic* variant) and centrifugal erythema (*panniculitic* variant). The characteristic pattern of inflammation with *lupus* on the skin is – in immunomorphological terms – known as "interface dermatitis," which is found at the junction of the dermis. The diagnostic value also involves anamnestic factors, particularly if onset occurs after exposure to sunlight: in *SLE* only a secondary venue, in *Lupus erythematosus* often the only clinical symptom.
  - *Discoid exanthem* mostly entails round, disc-like, centrally scarred red patches, often with characteristic desquamation, appearing on the trunk, shoulders, bottom, and upper legs. If there is a lack of systemic involvement it is classified as *discoid Lupus erythematosus*; exanthem can also appear with juvenile idiopathic arthritis (*JIA*).
  - *Orbita* with *red-blue-violet* and *livid* discoloration and edematous swelling of the upper lids (*periorbital edema, "lilac rings"*) and other parts of the body exposed to light (neck, hands, shoulders, extensor sides of the upper arms, back) – a diagnostic criterion of *PM/DM* (Fig. 94), may also be *SLE*.
- *Hands, extensor sides of arms, legs, and trunk*
  - Changes similar to *"butterfly rash"* are very typical
  - *Livedo reticularis or racemosa* (Figs. 2, 20a, 30–32) – persistent affectation of the skin on the trunk or extremities with violet, red, or blue reticular or mottled patterns, which are resistant to heat; regular circles are described as *Livedo reticularis*, irregular circles in a flash-like pattern as *Livedo racemosa* and occlusions of individual vessels with or without inflammation, come under *CTD, vasculitis, antiphospholipid* syndrome (APS), *livedoid vasculopathy*, and other diseases:
    - *Panarteritis nodosa*, a diagnostic criterion, Fig. 2
    - *Undifferentiated vasculitis* (CS 11)
    - *Antiphospholipid* syndrome (CS 6)
    - *Borreliosis* (CS 7), associated with disease activity
  - *Erythema* in the form of
    - Diffuse, poorly defined red patches in *CTD* (Figs. 27, 71)

- Multiple focal erythema in *sarcoidosis* (Fig. 90)
- Ring-like papules in *Granuloma annulare* (histologically similar to rheumatic nodules), DD *sarcoidosis* (Fig. 90)
- *Maculopapular exanthem (rash)*
  - *DM* "heliotropic exanthem" (Fig. 94) and *Gottron's* papules (on knuckles of the fingers, this location is atypical of *SLE*)
  - *Vasculitis* (Fig. 33, CS 12)
  - *Secondary vasculitis* with *RA* (Fig. 55)
  - *Still's* disease (in children/CS 66/and adult form/Fig. 131/)
  - Hypocomplementemic *urticarial vasculitis*
  - *Syphilis, secondary* (possible papulosquamous, pustular), distributed on the trunk (like to *Still's*, Fig. 131) and proximal extremities, involve the palms and soles (as in *pustular psoriasis*, Figs. 110–111ab)
- *Hemorrhagic diathesis* (cutaneous efflorescences, not displaceable, focal)
  - *Palpable purpura*, hemorrhagic type (Fig. 56a) or
  - Necrotizing ulcerating type/Fig. 56b/(with intrafocal bleeding)
  - *Petechiae* and *hemorrhagic purpura* (Fig. 78) with *thrombocytopenia*
  - *Purpura* with *hemorrhage, plaques,* and *epidermal necrolysis* (Figs. 110, 111b)

Common causes for *erythema* and *exanthem:*

- *Drug* and *contrast allergy* (*allergic vasculitis*, drug eruption, Figs. 110, 111ab)
- *Infections* and *tumors* (Chap. 5)
  - *Meningococcal sepsis*: here we see a combination of *purpura*, as in Fig. 56a, and *maculopapular exanthem*, as in Figs. 33, 90, 94, and 131
- Different systemic forms of *vasculitis: hypersensitivity vasculitis* and *Henoch–Schönlein* purpura (diagnostic criteria), in *Still's* disease (CS 66, Fig. 131), *cryoglobulinemic* vasculitis (a lead symptom, CS 20), and *Felty's* syndrome (CS 68)
- *Sarcoidosis* (Figs. 83, 90)

Further efflorescences in such localization:

- Raised erythematous plaques with nodules and pustules, at the same time *fever, arthralgia, episcleritis* (*Sweet* syndrome, often paraneoplastic)
- *Urticaria* in the form of *wheals* (*C1-inhibitor deficiency*) and/or *hematomas* centrally, if they persist for more than 24 h (in hypocomplementary *hypersensitivity vasculitis*, Figs. 56ab or *drug reaction*, Figs. 110, 111b)
- *Photodermatitis* (*urticaria, bullous changes* following exposure to sunlight, highly specific to *SLE*)
- *Exfoliative dermatitis* as an expression of *Stevens–Johnson* syndrome (*SJS*) affected the whole body in *SLE* (*bullous LE*) in the form of scalded skin or *Lyell's* syndrome with *epidermolysis* (extreme variant of *SJS*), with fatal outcome (in our observational case), more often drug-induced (e.g., MMF/CellCept®) or immunologically mediated reactions to exogenous factors (e.g., herpes virus)

- *Erythema migrans* in *borreliosis* (a stage I diagnostic criterion)
- *Lymphadenosis cutis benigna*, as in Fig. 20a, in *borreliosis* (morphologically no *vasculitis!*)
- *Nail fold* (painful reddening, calcification, hyperkeratoses, infarcts, *teleangiectasis*) in primary and secondary *vasculitis*/Fig. 71/, but also in *psoriasis* (Fig. 15a)

9.1.2
Ulcerations, Gangrene, or Scarring

in:

- *Necrotizing vasculitis* of the *medium-sized arteries* with *thrombosis* (Figs. 2, 30–31, 55, 101a, 132) or *livedoid vasculitis* represent a combination of vasculopathy with intravascular thrombosis (possible in Figs. 30–31)
  - Only with *panarteritis nodosa* (Figs. 10–11), hence such a pattern – our own observation 30 years ago – is not a condition but a diagnosis
  - Not to such an extent even in secondary *vasculitis* (*MCTD*, Fig. 71), *antiphospholipid* syndrome,
  - *Cryoglobulinemic* vasculitis with *benign monoclonal gammapathy* (Fig. 132)
  - Also possible with *giant cell arteritis* and blindness
  - *Rheumatoid vasculitis* (Figs. 55, 101a)

Such fatal changes occurred in association with systemic *vasculitis*; less dramatic changes are to be viewed as a gateway to *infections* (sepsis).

- *Acral, necrotizing skin lesions* and digital ischemia (Figs. 14, 47, 113)
  - *SSc* (CS 16, 54)
  - *MCTD*
  - Drug-induced *vasculitis* (CS 42)
  - *Peripheral arterial* (CS 4) or *venous disease*
  - *Aortoiliac occlusive disease* may manifest by atheroembolism to the foot in the "blue toe" or "trash foot" syndrome
  - *Takayasu arteriitis* (own observations as in Fig. 113; aside from "pulseless disease," distal gangrene is extremely uncommon; in this case, the contributing cofactors/cryoglobulinemia, ACLA/play an important role)
  - *Thromboangiitis obliterans*/Buerger's disease/as Fig. 47 (digital gangrene without the evidence of internal organ involvement, often with a migratory thrombophlebitis)
  - *Thromboembolism,* for example, APS, infective endocarditis
  - *Nail fold infarcts* in seropositive *RA* (Bywaters' lesion)
  - Triggered and intensified by cold (in *cryoglobulinemic* vasculitis)
  - *Paraneoplasia* (Chap. 5)
  - Squamous cell carcinoma, for example, within scars, and, less often, melanoma
  - Infections, for example, ecthyma, caused by streptococcus

- Hemoglobinopathies or hereditary spherocytosis
- Cholesterol emboly
- DD with necrosis in diabetic *polyneuropathy*
- *Genital ulcers*, for example, in the form of balanitis (*ReA, Behçet's* disease)
- *Pyoderma gangrenosum* (idiopathic or in immunosuppressed patients, most commonly associated disorders are *ulcerative colitis* and *Crohn's* disease, less commonly *chronic active hepatitis*, seropositive *RA*, in a similar form to Fig. 55, or *myeloproliferative disorders, benign monoclonal gammopathy,* and *chronic recurrent multifocal osteomyelitis [CRMO]*)

9.1.3
Pustules, Sterile (Pseudofolliculitis), Papulopustular Lesions

Acne, vulgaris pustules or nodules, pyoderma, associated with

- *Psoriasis vulgaris pustulosa* (Figs. 15, 110, 111a, 129b)
- *Arthritis* or *dactylitis* in *PsA, ReA, SAPHO* syndrome (Figs. 65ab)
- Drug induced by TNF therapy (CS 41)
- *Behçet's* disease (CS 26), *Sweet* syndrome (also raised erythematous plaques or nodules)
- *Toxic pustuloderma* (drug reaction)
- *Staphylococcal pyoderma*
- *PAPA* syndrome (acne, pyoderma gangrenosum, pyogenic arthritis)
- *Subcorneal pustulosis* (*Sneddon-Wilkinson* syndrome)
- *Gonococcal* infection and *syphilis, secondary* (pustules on palms and soles)

9.1.4
Induration and Tightening of the Skin

Induration and tightening of the skin is an expression of increased connective tissue or the *sclerotic* processes underway therein and in the vessels. This can be easily proven by capillary microscopy (known as a *scleroderma*-typical capillary microscopic pattern).

A distinction is made between the following clinical forms of such processes:

- *Scleroderma (diffuse cutaneous systemic sclerosis)*, a primary criterion of *SSc*, developing in three consecutive stages:
  - *Edema* usually non-pitting and painless in the form of *"puffy hands"* (Fig. 130c or as in Fig. 7); this brief phase of exudative inflammation is particularly suited to antiinflammatory therapy
  - *Induration* with dermal thickening and epidermal thinning or proliferative inflammation (a target for immunosuppression), as in Figs. 47, 52; a rapid rate of skin thickness is associated with an increased frequency and earlier appearance of organ involvement
  - *Fibrosis* and *atrophy* (skin folds difficult to lift, Fig. 18)

Such changes can mostly be found on the

- Arms (above the wrists)
- Face (*microstomia*-perioral fibrosis with *"purse-string mouth"* and pinched nose)
- Trunk ("growth in carapace" – a poor prognostic factor)
- *Sclerodactyly* or *acroscleroderma (limited cutaneous systemic sclerosis)* limited to the fingers, possibly with *calcinosis* (Fig. 18), and toes
  - Acral thickening, hand (skin between MCP joints and wrist), particularly on the dorsal side of the fingers, scar-like changes, necrosis and loss of tissue at the tips of the fingers, *rat-bite necrosis* (Fig. 47)
  - Tapered *"Madonna fingers," contractures* (Figs. 18, 130c)
- *Morphea, linear scleroderma,* and *en coup de sabre,* that is, localized scleroderma, in most cases *localized* (one or a few lesions) or in some patients *generalized* (widespread cutaneous lesions without systemic involvement)
- *Buschke scleroderma* (deposition of dermal mucopolysaccharide in the form of symmetrical indurated skin most on neck extending to face and upper limbs, associated with streptococcal infection, diabetes, and paraproteinemia)
- *Pseudoscleroderma* or *Scleroderma mimickers* is not associated with *Raynaud's* phenomenon (here lie a difference for *SSc*) and characterized by similar changes in
  - *Osteoarthritis* (Fig. 130a), *RA*
  - Thoracic outlet syndrome
  - *Scleromyxedema* (involves the head and neck rather than the extremities, possible presence of a paraprotein)
  - *Diabetes mellitus* (diabetic cheiroarthropathy)
  - Drugs (e.g., cisplatin, bleomycin, sympathomimetics)
  - Chemicals (polyvinyl chloride, silicone, mammaplasty)
  - *Paraneoplastic* (in fasciitis, Fig. 95), in *carcinoid* syndrome
  - Primary *amyloidosis*
  - Chronic *graft-versus-host* reaction
  - Chronic renal insufficiency (*nephrogenic systemic fibrosis* possibly with chitin formation and fibrotic changes in the lungs, muscles, heart, and esophagus, strongly associated with gadolinium exposure)
- (Eosinophilic) *fasciitis* (Fig. 95), *eosinophilia-myalgia* syndrome

9.1.5
Aphthae, Aphthous Stomatitis

Aphthae, aphthous stomatitis/Fig. 76/(but also ulcerations in the region of the genitals and colon) are to be seen to some extent as *vasculitic* changes in the *small vessels* and appear in the form of recurrent, "open wounds": a diagnostic criterion (also with scarring) and a *sign of activity* (upon recurrence) in *SLE* (painless), but also *Behçet's* (CS 26), *SLE* (CS 64), *Wegener's,* other forms of *vasculitis,* and MTX *mucositis* (in the setting of the MTX therapy).

9.1.6
Alopecia

Alopecia diffusa or seldom *areata* (Fig. 82) is a sign of *vasculitis* of the small vessels (a diagnostic criterion for *SLE*, CS 29), on recurrence a *sign of activity* (completely reversible by glucocorticoid therapy), which could be the case with *PM/DM, SSc, iron deficiency, thyroid dysfunction*, due to medication, *stress*, localized and generalized *infections* (e.g., *syphilis, secondary* with *mucocutaneous* lesions and generalized *lymphadenopathy*).

9.2
Blood Vessels

The type of vessel and nature of the *pathophysiological* changes in the affected vessels are important.[13] Direct vascular involvement can be categorized into *three mega syndromes* by clinical examination and imaging (Doppler sonography, angiography, MRI, PET, capillaroscopy):

A. *Inflammatory syndromes in*:

9.2.1
Small Vessels with Cutaneous Efflorescences

(See Chap. 9.1)

9.2.2
Direct Inflammatory Changes in Medium and Large Vessels

- *Tissue degeneration* (Chap. 9.1.2):
  - *Ulceration* (Figs. 2, 10–11, 30–31, 55, 71, 101a)
  - *Scarring* (Figs. 32, 101b)
  - Peripheral *gangrene* with *rat-bite necrosis* (Figs. 47, 113)
  - *Aphthae*, mucosal ulcerations (Fig. 76)
  - Necrotizing (accompanying tissue damage) *purpura*
- *Thrombotic conditions*
  - *Thrombophlebitis* or *phlebothrombosis* (*SLE*, CS 34), *Behçet's* disease (first vascular event is deep vein thrombosis of the legs)
  - *Trousseau's* syndrome in *paraneoplasia* (Chap. 5)
  - *Thromboangiitis obliterans* (*Buerger's* disease), involving small- and medium-sized arteries and veins in the distal upper and lower extremities
- *Narrowing or stenosis or irregularities in the intima* of the aorta or other large vessels (Ultrasound and more likely MRI finding and angiography) in

- *Takayasu* (Fig. 77a) and *giant-cell arteritis* (nodular thickening of the temporal artery and diplopia on physical examination is extremely helpful when present), *polymyalgia rheumatica*
- *Aortoiliac occlusive disease* in patients with peripheral arterial disease and involvement of the infrarenal aorta and iliac arteries; aortitis may result from vasculitis in the *vasa vasorum* of the adventitia (Chap. 9.2.5)
- *Behçet's* disease with subsequent arterial occlusions (CS 26) associated with inflammatory venous thromboses
- *Cogan's* syndrome associated with ocular inflammation and audiovestibular dysfunction
- *Relapsing polychondritis* (aortitis)
- *Sarcoidosis* (aortitis)
- *IgG4*-related systemic disease (aortitis)
- *Infections* (syphilis, tuberculosis)
- *Palpable nodes* (Figs. 33, 109, → Chaps. 3.2.1 and 9.4.2) in
  - *Panarteritis, microscopic* (Fig. 33) or *nodosa* (along the mesenterial arteries or subcutaneous)
  - *Erythema nodosum* (CS 40)
  - *Sweet* syndrome, no vasculitis in the strict sense (reddish nodules, later sterile *pustules* and *vesicles* on the scalp, neck, and upper extremities)
- *Aneurysms,* measuring up to 1 cm in the aorta, visceral arteries, kidneys, liver, with stenosis (thoracic aortic aneurysms confirmed by annual chest radiographs and angiography) in
  - *Giant-cell arteritis* (often several years after the diagnosis)
  - *Panarteritis nodosa* (most microaneurysms within blood vessels in the mesenteric and renal vasculature)
  - *Behçet's* disease (most pulmonary arteries aneurysm)
  - *Sepsis lenta* (in our case developed the palpable *micotic aneurysm* on the *A. femoralis* as the first clinical signs)
  - Genetic disorders (*Marfan's* and *Ehlers–Danlos* syndrome)
- *Focal changes* (lesions of *"white matter"*) in the *CNS* (specifically determined by MRI, Fig. 50), in *CNS* vasculitis (CS 18, 72, → Chap. 10.6)
- *Enhancements* in the ascending aorta as well as in the supraaortic vessels and (peri) vascular structures on PET:
  - *Takayasu's arteritis* (CS 25, Figs. 74, 77b)
  - *Giant-cell arteritis,* in some cases of the *polymyalgia rheumatica*
  - *Periaortitis*, for example, associated with *Ormond's* disease (can also be detected by CT and MRI)
- *Audiovestibular* dysfunction and sensorineural *hearing loss* (rather indirect inflammatory changes in medium vessels in *giant-cell arteritis* and other vasculitides → Chap. 10.9.3).
- *Positive biopsy* of temporal arteries is the gold standard for diagnosing *giant-cell arteritis*; it may only be positive in 30–40% of patients; the false-negative rate is approximately 10%.

B. Ischemic syndrome resulting from *stenosis* or *occlusion* of the blood vessel and cause various kinds of vascular insufficiency:

9.2.3
Raynaud Phenomenon

Raynaud phenomenon results from exaggerated vascular response to cold temperatures or stress. It is a sign of arterial vasoconstriction and/or stenosis (Figs. 14, 47, 52, 113) and could be (sub) acute (CS 16) or exist for many years in monosymptomatic form as a vasospastic episode with transient digital ischemia without trophic skin changes, for example, in young women (*primary* syndrome, in more than 90% of all cases), or precede other diseases (*secondary* syndrome). The *primary* form occurs in the absence of any associated disease or a definable cause for the attacks. Typical in such cases are: no evidence of tissue gangrene or digital pitting, no abnormal nail fold capillary microscopy and negative ANA, not to require treatment. Its severity could vary in all forms of *secondary* syndrome by *CTD* and *vasculitis*.

Clinical

- Age of onset >40 years, males presenting at any age
- Specific discoloration: clearly defined white-red-blue discoloration, cyanosis (white and/or blue attack) of the fingers and sometimes also the toes (reactive vasodilation)/ Fig. 52/, pain associated with attacks
- Pitted scars (Fig. 101b) or degeneration of finger pulp, "*rat-bite necrosis*" (an ACR criterion for *SSc*) or of a finger "*sausage finger*" (DD *PsA*, Fig. 15a)
- Affecting the fingers (Figs. 18, 52, 130c), toes, nasal apex, auricles; often *swelling* of digits affected, digital pulp loss in the fingertips and a calcium deposit in the pulp of the finger (Fig. 18)
- Abnormal nail fold capillary (in contrast to primary phenomenon)
- Stable and at the same time episodic, induced by exposure to cold/damp, emotional stress
- Positive ANA (Chap. 11.1)

Etiology Varies

- *Rheumatological causes*
  - *SSc* (Fig. 18, CS 16, 19, 54) and other forms of *CTD* and *vasculitis*
  - Stenosis of the large vessels within the scope of *vasculitis* (Fig. 61)
  - *Cryoglobulinemic vasculitis* (hepatitis C, with 80–90% positivity for anti-HCV-Ab)
- *Arteriosclerosis obliterans,* that is, occlusive arterial disease (CS 4)
- Mechanical causes
  - Thoracic outlet syndrome, neurovascular changes around the shoulder girdle
  - Cervical rib (most unilateral evidence of vascular insufficiency)
  - Vascular embolus or occlusion
  - Vibration injury

- Drug induced (antidepressants/CS 42/, hormone contraceptives, bleomycin, vinblastin, beta-blockers, ergotamine)
- Neurological disorders (migraine headaches)
- Hematological disorders (with paraproteins, cold agglutinins, polycythemia)
- Neoplasias (paraneoplasia → Chap. 5)
- Endocrine disorders (hypothyroidism, pheochromocytoma, carcinoid syndrome)

9.2.4
Acrosclerosis or Osteolysis

Acrosclerosis or osteolysis (clinical, Figs. 18, 47 and radiological sign, Fig. 23) of the terminal phalanges is indicative, if the two syndromes collide, of advanced forms of *Raynaud's* syndrome and arterial circulatory disorders with luminal narrowing, most commonly in *SSc* (as secondary criteria) or vasculitis of the *medium-sized vessels (panarteritis nodosa, Buerger's* disease/thrombangiitis obliterans/, *hypersensitivity vasculitis*) or a *bone tumor (primary* or *secondary)* or a *stress fracture*/Fig. 54/or chronic recurrent multifocal osteomyelitis (*CRMO*). *Acrosclerosis* is defined as a component of *CREST* syndrome.

9.2.5
Intermittent, Arterial, Spinal, Jaw Claudication, and Aortoiliac Disease

Claudicatio intermittens of the extremities (CS 4) mostly appear as the classical form in *Arteriosclerosis obliterans* with load-dependent pain as well as in vasculitis (*Buerger's* disease). The same pattern quickly following the initiation of chewing – *jaw claudication* – is to be seen in the masticatory muscles with *Takayasu's* and *giant-cell arteritis*. With the exception of vascular problems this could, in the event of massive *spinal canal stenosis*, take the form of *Claudicatio spinalis*, which can be reversed completely by surgery. Pain-free manifestation is extremely rare (*Claudicatio arteriosa*) in subacute stenosis of the *Aorta abdominalis*, that is, *Leriche's* syndrome within the context of *aortoiliac disease* (as result of thrombosis in aorta/Fig. 12/expressed by severe weakness in the legs and enabling "just a few steps" and "no strength in the legs," CS 3).

Pay attention with this syndrome to:

- New onset of the syndrome should be interpreted as a *sign of activity*
- Duration of more than 6 months should be considered as *damage*

Leriche's syndrome can present within the context of *aortoiliac occlusion* or *aortoiliac disease* (how to describe it at the moment) itself, not only in *subacute* (CS 3, Fig. 12) but also in *acute forms* (Fig. 132), as result of

(a) *Thrombosis*
- In the bifurcation of the aorta from *antiphospholipid* syndrome/Fig. 12/
- In a preexisting, severely narrowed segment of the aorta.[7]

In our case, for visual diagnosis/Fig.132/, the patient has systemic vasculitis associated with cryoglobulinemia and benign monoclonal gammopathy leading to acute gangrene in the upper third of both thighs. In fact, in the angiography of the abdominal aorta, the pelvic and leg vessels (present) show a normal aorta and pelvic vessels, but absolute ischemia in the medium and small vessels of the legs. Histologically, the amputated legs reveal vasculitis in these vessels with endothelial proliferations and thrombosis. The question was: How to explain the strict symmetry of the demarcation line and vessel infestation? It is better explained expressly as *selective occlusions* of the medium and small vessels of the legs as a result of *in situ* thrombosis and endothelial proliferation, *in a preexisting, severely narrowed segment of the aorta*, possibly with vasculitis in the *vasa vasorum* of the adventitia

(b) *Massive embolism* in the bifurcation of the aorta (a classical form)

(c) *Atheroembolism* in the foot within the context of *aortoiliac occlusive disease* in a patient with peripheral arterial disease.

9.2.6
Pulse and Blood Pressure Differences

(With large vessel involvement)

- Blood pressure difference
  - More than 10 mmHg between the two arms (*vasculitis*, see below)
  - More than 20 mmHg between the arms and legs (*aortic coarctation*)
- Pulse difference and minimization, possible *absence of a pulse* in the *A. radialis, carotis, brachialis, femoralis, tibialis posterior, dorsalis pedis* (*arteriosclerosis obliterans, vasculitis*, and *Behçet's* disease, *aortic coarctation* above all *Takayasu*/has been termed "pulseless disease"/also applies to *giant-cell arteritis*, and *Buerger's* disease)

A morphological substrate of such symptoms is shown in Figs. 12, 61.

9.2.7
Aortic Arch Syndrome

Aortic arch syndrome (Fig. 61) is described as *Takayasu's arteritis* and is induced by inflammatory *intima* and *media proliferation* (*giant-cell arteritis*) of the aorta, the outlets at the aortic arch and pulmonary arteries. The same histology can be found for the medium-calibre peripheral arteries in *giant-cell arteritis* with or without *polymyalgia rheumatica*, and the same clinical findings also in *arteriosclerosis obliterans, thromboses*, and *neoplasias*.

The following *stenotic symptoms* may occur:

- *Claudicatio* symptoms of the upper extremities on exertion (involvement of the outlets at the aortic arch)

- Pain in the face, jaw, and tongue (in our case, the earlier diagnosis of *giant-cell arteritis* was identified by a dentist, who, in a patient with mandibular edema, detected palpable thickened *A. sublingualis*; the biopsy of the *A. temporalis* performed subsequently was negative)
- *Vertigo* and *impaired vision* on involvement of the *A. carotis and A. centralis retinae*
- Reduced pulses in one or both brachial arteries
- Pulse difference between both *carotid arteries*
- Blood pressure difference between both arms (see above)
- Auscultation difference and stenotic sounds over the *Aorta abdominalis, Aa. brachial, subclavian, and axillary* (*Takayasu* and *giant-cell arteritis*)
- Arteriographic *constriction* or *occlusion* of the whole aorta, its main branches (Fig. 61) or of large arteries of the upper and lower extremities

The following syndromes may round off the above mentioned symptoms:

- *Arterial hypertension* on involvement or stenosis of the *A. renalis*
- *Pneumonitis* on involvement of the pulmonary arteries (Chap. 10.2.3)
- Tender and pulse-free *temporal arteries* (in *giant-cell arteritis, polymyalgia rheumatica*)
- *Mononeuritis multiplex* (Chap. 9.7.2)

C. *Noninflammatory syndromes*

9.2.8
Teleangiectasis

Teleangiectasis affecting the entire body and mucous membranes, noninflammatory vascular changes (often associated with primary *biliary liver cirrhosis* (e.g., *CREST* syndrome), also *PM* (on nail fold and skin), *SSc*, *SLE* (over the focal margin of lesions in *discoid lupus*), *MCTD*. In the case of ectatic superficial cutaneous and mucosal vessels, consideration must be given to *Fabry's* disease.

9.2.9
Thrombosis (Venous and Arterial) and Thromboembolisms

in:

- *Primary* (*Sneddon's* syndrome)/CS 3 and 6/and *secondary* (all forms of *CTD*) *antiphospholipid* syndrome (Chap. 11.4)
- *Trousseau's* syndrome as paraneoplasia (Chap. 5)
- *Peripheral occlusions* (*giant-cell* and *Takayasu's arteritis*)
- *Venous thrombotic events* (*Wegener's* and probably other ANCA-associated vasculitides have this predisposition)
- *Thrombophlebitis*, superficial, also in the region of the portal system and superior vena cava (*Behçet's* disease)

- *Thrombangiitis* in the form of *migratory superficial venous thrombophlebitis* (*Buerger's* disease)
- *Thrombophilia* (coagulation difficulties)
- *Peripheral gangrene*
  - Of all toes in *Endocarditis verrucosa* (own observation in a female patient with *rheumatic fever*)
  - With *cholesterol embolisms* (individual fingers)
  - *Septic thromboses* (bacterial or candidal *sepsis*)
  - *Takayasu's arteritis, Buerger's* disease

9.2.10
Erythromelalgia

Erythromelalgia is regarded as a syndrome of paroxysmal vasodilation.

Clinical

- Attacks of burning pain, redness, and high skin temperature on the feet and less often on the hands (in our case was associated with *small fiber neuropathy*, see Chap. 9.7.1).
- It is important to distinguish the rare *primary* forms from common *secondary* forms.
- The underlying diseases are of a rheumatological nature (*SLE, RA, Sudeck's* syndrome, *panniculitis*) or associated with *paraneoplasia* (preceding a *myeloproliferative* syndrome by some years).

9.3
Joints and Periarticular Structures

(See also Chap. 1)
  Articular involvement is characterized by the aforementioned syndromes and could in principle occur in all forms of *CTD* and *vasculitis*. The distinction lies, thereby, in the *absence of pannus formation*. The following clinical and radiological features emerge:

9.3.1
Arthralgia

- *Very common, but unstable*
- Stable *arthralgia* (e.g., throughout the day) should be ascribed to *arthritis*
- Often *very intensive*, but certainly disproportionate to objective joint status (possible involvement of *tendons/fasciae* or *aseptic necrosis* (Fig. 121) or *Fabry's* disease)
- Combined with *myalgia* (also in *undifferentiated CTD* and *vasculitis*)

9.3.2
Arthritis

Arthritis, in fact all reported types (Chap. 1.3), in all forms of *CTD* and *vasculitis*, could also be consistent with *RA* (Fig. 70). The main differences are:

- Mostly *non-erosive* (Fig. 72) and *unstable*
- Seldom *erosive* changes (cannot be diagnosed by X-ray, but by MRI), very rarely involving joint deformities and *mutilations*
- *Periarticular fibrosis* (Fig. 128c), not tender in such a case
- Seldom *polyarthritis* (e.g., *SLE, CREST* syndrome), mostly *oligoarthritis* (*CTD* and *vasculitis)*
- Often *oligosymptomatic*, possibly with *pleural involvement* (a variant of chronic *SLE*)
- When associated with *myalgia, PM,* other forms of *CTD* and *vasculitis* must not be overlooked

9.3.3
Contractures

(As in Figs. 5, 42, 43, 62, 63, 70, 80, 104, 129c, 130a)

- Joint-related *(arthrogenic)*, painful (due to *inflammatory arthritis,* e.g., in *SLE*) and painless (due to *sclerotic* changes and *calcinosis* of the periarticular structures in *SSc,* Fig. 18)
- *Muscular, fascial, and neurological* in *MCTD* (Fig. 70, CS 24, serious malpositioning was described as *Jaccoud's* arthropathy), *PM,* flexion contractures of the hands in *fasciitis* (Fig. 95), *paraplegia* (Fig. 19)

9.3.4
Luxations, Subluxations, Deviations

Luxations, subluxations, and deviations result from damage to the ligament apparatus (as in Figs. 5/thumbs/, 42, 43, 59, 70, 72, 104, MCP, 122c – status following corrective surgery).

Such changes are seen in particular with *SLE, MCTD* (Fig. 70) and are difficult to differentiate from those specific to *RA*. The presence of erosions and their severity is pivotal, and in the case of *CTD* they are visible radiologically only in exceptional cases (but more often on MRI). These non-erosive changes with deformities are also known as Jaccoud's arthritis. *Mutilations* and spontaneous *osteolysis* are rare in *SSc, SLE,* but more common in *RA, PsA,* and *JIA.*

9.4
Subcutis and Fasciae

(See Chaps. 3.2 and 3.7) could also be affected in the event of *CTD* and *vasculitis*.

9.4.1
Panniculitis

Panniculitis is an inflammation of the fatty tissue and may be associated with *vasculitis* in *SLE, MCTD, SSc*, presenting with

- *Diffuse*, non-nodular *forms* (*Lupus profundus*, Figs. 27, 71), vivid, hardly differing at all from *erysipelas*, often treated with antibiotics, responding well to glucocorticoids (CS 24, 34), and regarded as a consequence of *secondary vasculitis*; DD with *Weber–Christian* disease (acute nodular panniculitis, e.g., fat necrosis) without (e.g., trauma) or with (e.g., CTD, pancreatic disease, lypodystrophy) systemic disease , *leukemic infiltrates, paraneoplasias.*
- *Erythema nodosum* in the form of subcutaneous nodules (Fig. 109) may also be seen with *vasculitis* (*Takayasu's arteritis, Churg–Strauss* syndrome, *Behçet's* disease, *lethal midline granuloma*), *Granuloma annulare* and *sarcoidosis.*
- Another form of granulomatous inflammation in *sarcoidosis* is shown in Figs. 83 and 90.

9.4.2
Nodules

Nodules (see Chap. 3.1) may present in two ways:

- *Painful*, palpable cutaneously and subcutaneously/Fig. 33/, as a combination of vasculitic and aneurysmatic changes (*microscopic polyangiitis*, CS 12) or fat necrosis or generalized lipodystrophy.
- *Painless*, more papulous changes on the extensor sides of the fingers (*Gottron's sign*) in *PM/DM*. DD *rheumatoid nodules* (Figs. 3, 104) and *lupus erythema* (affects the areas between the small joints of the fingers and spares the knuckles), *Erythema induratum Bazin, panniculitic* T-cell and B-cell *lymphoma.*
- *Churg–Strauss* and *Wegener's* syndrome often associated with high level of the rheumatoid factors (CS 72); in these cases cutaneous extravascular necrotizing granulomas (typically for both diseases) can be mistaken clinically and pathologically for rheumatoid nodules.

9.4.3
Calcinosis Subcutis (Thibierge-Weissenbach Syndrome)

Calcinosis subcutis (Fig. 18) consisting of *calcium phosphate or calcium apatite*

- Presenting with solitary, white-colored, painless *cutaneous nodes* on the fingers, elbows
- Prevails in *CREST* syndrome (CS 32), then in *SSc* (Fig. 18), *PM, SLE*

9.4.4
Eosinophilic Fasciitis (Shulman's Syndrome)

Eosinophilic fasciitis presenting as scleroderma-like syndrome with involvement of the dermis, subcutis, and deep fasciae in *two forms:*

- *Primary* as an entity
  - *Arthralgia/myalgia* syndrome
  - *Scleroderma*-type induration of the skin, mostly on the hands, forearms, possibly with swelling, tenderness
  - *Carpal tunnel* syndrome and *flexion contractures* (Fig. 95) of the hands
  - Neither *organ involvement* nor *Raynaud's* syndrome
- *Secondary* in association with
  - *SSc* with specific organ involvement
  - Drug-induced (tuberculostatics, H2 blocker cimetidine)

9.5
Tendons, Tendon Sheaths, and Ligaments

Tendomyotic symptoms (Chap. 3.4) may arise during the many months of the prodromal stage or during the *course* of any form of *vasculitis* (e.g., *microscopic polyangiitis*) or *CTD*. The following are typical:

- *Tenosynovitis* of the extensor tendons of the hand (*swan-neck deformity, ulnar deviation* of long fingers from *(sub) luxation* (Figs. 70, 95, 104) with or without (Fig. 72) minimal *erosions*
- *Tenosynovitis, drug-induced* (glucocorticoids, antibiotics)
- Damage to the *ligament apparatus* is seen mostly with *CTD* due to deviations (Fig. 70) and periarticular fibrosis (Fig. 128c), resembling proliferative *arthritis* (Fig. 63) and thus complicating local diagnosis
- *Fibrosis* of the tendon sheath or adjacent tissues (often with *SSc*), *tendon ruptures* should be regarded as a consequence of inflammation (*damage*)
- *Enthesopathy* in *Behçet's* disease (associated with acne and arthritis)
- *Carpal tunnel* syndrome (often with *SSc*)

9.6
Muscles

This multitude of important syndromes should primarily be viewed from a pathophysiological standpoint, by considering the possibility of a *non-inflammatory (fibromyalgia, myodystrophy,* endocrine and drug-induced *myopathy*→ Chaps. 3.4, 3.5) or *inflammatory (myositis) myopathies.* At the same time it is important to differentiate between *primary (PM/DM)* and *secondary (RA, vasculitis* or *CTD)* forms of *myositis,* which can be manifested in the following syndromes:

9.6.1
Myalgia

Myalgia of an inflammatory nature is used to describe stubborn (due to muscular ischemia) *muscular pain,* mostly in the calves (*SLE, MCTD, panarteritis nodosa, undifferentiated vasculitis, thromboangiitis obliterans,* and *eosinophilic fasciitis*). Serious, persistent shoulder-neck pain with restricted mobility (patient often reliant on outside help) and tenderness is typical of *polymyalgia rheumatica.* When accompanied by eosinophilia, but no organ involvement, the myalgia is described as *eosinophilia-myalgia* syndrome.

9.6.2
Myositis

Myositis is a syndrome involving *muscular inflammation* with exudative, proliferative, granulomatous and necrotic changes in the muscles.

Clinically it presents, above all, in the form of *myasthenia, muscular atrophy,* and *myalgia.*

It is important, thereby, to establish the *emphasis* of the *involvement,* as follows:

- *Proximal myasthenia, symmetrical, progressive,* with or without *myalgia,* with *muscular atrophy,* affecting the upper and lower extremities as well as the trunk in terms of everyday mobility as far as *pareses.* Such symptoms are to be viewed as an expression
  - Of *highly active* myositic and/or dystrophic changes in *sub-/acute PM/DM* (primary diagnostic criterion), *MCTD* (CS 24)
  - or even *myopathies:*
  - *Drug-induced* (glucocorticoids, statins, clofibrate, DMARDs, e.g., chloroquine, cyclosporine, D penicillamine, colchicine) or
  - *Toxic* (alcohol, illegal drugs, e.g., ecstasy) or
  - *Endocrine* (hypo-/hyperthyroidism)
- *Distal myasthenia* of the extremities, mostly *asymmetrical* with fine motor deficits, indicative of *inclusion body myositis*

- *Myasthenic* syndrome could be *fibromyalgia* (32-year-old female presented in a wheelchair); if there is a lack of evidence of *thymoma* on chest CT and of acetylcholine receptor antibodies, *myasthenia* can virtually be ruled out
- In the case of *muscular atrophy, cerebrovascular events and spinal cord injury* (Fig. 19) must be ruled out
- *Amyotrophy, intercostal* (as with *RA* in Figs. 5, 35, 42, 58, 80, 104, 129c, also with *SLE, MCTD*/Fig. 70/, *SSc*/Fig. 18/), is also to be regarded as a consequence of *myositis*
- In the event of *myalgia*, consideration is to be given not only to the rare *PM*, but also to *common polymyalgia rheumatica*, if everything (age group, localization, *arthritis*) adds up
- *Ocular myositis* mostly affects the outer muscles of the eyes (cortisone-dependent pain in the eye region, convergence disorders, double vision)
- Laryngeal musculature (*dysphonia*), which is distinguished from *progressive muscular dystrophy*, whereby the laryngeal, pharyngeal, and neck muscles are not affected
- Esophageal musculature (*dysphagia*)
- Heart (signs of *myocarditis*: dyspnea, tachycardia, cardiac irregularity)
- Muscles and fasciae of the hands, elbows (*muscle contractures*)

9.6.3
Muscular Calcinosis

Muscular calcinosis occurs, in the same way as *subcutaneous calcinosis* (Chap. 9.4.3), due to calcium deposits in the musculature of the extremities, and could be

- *Primary* (*Myosits calcificans*) or
- *Secondary* as a result of inflammatory and dystrophic processes (*PM*)

9.6.4
CK Elevation

CK elevation (CS 54) is a valuable test *initially* for diagnosing *PM/DM* or *myositis* associated with other forms of *CTD* (*SSc, MCTD*), and then for monitoring therapy.
    Thereby, the following should be considered:

- *CK* elevation may correlate with the degree of muscle inflammation rather *early* in the course of the disease as opposed to *later* when muscle athrophy is more likely
- *CK* elevation could also, in noninflammatory *muscular dystrophies*, result from, for example,
    - Thyroid dysfunction (CS 54), and is greatly influenced partly by muscle bulk, by any muscle strain or exercise occurring shortly beforehand

- Inherited group of progressive myopathic disorders (distinguished from PM by the positive family history, relatively early onset and slow progression)
- *CK* elevation is often accompanied by increases in *CK-MB* (thus the question of cardiac involvement arises), liver enzymes (*GOT, GPT, LDH*), *aldolase* in the blood, as well as *myoglobin*, also in the urine
- *CK-MB* elevation could be disproportionately high in
  - Acute *myocardial infarction*
  - *Myositis of the eye muscles* (up to 65% in one female patient aged 38 with cortisone-dependent eye pain)
  - *Sarcoid myopathy*
  - *Muscle trauma* or physical overload even with extensive training or following intramuscular injections
  - *Infectious* (bacterial) *myositis*, for example, with abscess in the jaw area (our observation) or in HIV
  - *Drug-induced myopathy,* for example, long-term use of *statins*: an 82-year-old male with ischemic heart disease (taking 20 mg simvastatin for 10 years) experienced episodes of extreme myasthenia which "was better" after stopping the medication. Lab findings (at that time the patient had no *myalgia* or *myasthenia*): CK (628 U/L; normal <190), CK-MB (1171 U/L; normal <25), CK-MB% (186%; normal <6%); *acute myocardial infarction* and *PM/DM* were largely ruled out
- Normal *CK* values should be regarded as
  - *Discriminatory* in the first potential disease (*polymyalgia rheumatica*)
  - *Typical* of *inclusion body myositis*, but *PM/DM* is not ruled out
  - *Normal serum CK* by *active myositis* is more likely in *DM* that in *PM* (rather unlikely in this setting)
  - *Untypical* with an episode in correlation to therapy, particularly with *cortisone*
  - Possibly *paraneoplastic*

9.7
Nerves (Peripheral)

Such involvement (Chap. 3.12.2) is regarded as *vasculitis neuropathy* or *Vasa nervorum vasculitis*, and characterized by neurological deficits or losses (motoric and/or sensory), which are best documented by extensive neurological consultation. Here, it is important to first rule out compression or thrombotic processes. Such a syndrome is most likely *vasculitis induced*, and has been seen in *all forms* of *CTD* and *vasculitis* with varying frequencies and severities, and thus no *nosological distinctions* could be made due to this syndrome. In this case only the correlations and staging diagnostics (Chap. 13) could be help.

The sensory neuropathy appearing from an *autoimmune disease* has different types, for example, distal symmetric polyneuropathy, sensory mononeuritis multiplex, small fiber neuropathy.

9.7.1
Polyneuropathy

Sensomotoric (CS 18, 48) with severe pain and weakness in the extremities or a lack of muscle extension reflexes is attributable to the involvement of the *Vasa* Vasorum of the peripheral nervous system and mostly seen in:

- *CTD (juvenile Sjögren's* syndrome/CS 18/, *SLE, MCTD)*
- *RA*/rheumatoid vasculitis/(Figs. 100, 101)
- *Vasculitis (Churg–Strauss* syndrome/CS 72/, *Wegener's,* and *hypersensitivity vasculitis*/Fig. 113/, but not in *Behçet's* disease
- *Vasculitis neuropathy* must be differentiated from other types of neuropathy:
- *Diabetic* polyneuropathies, possibly with *ulcerations*
- *Restless legs* syndrome (a sensorimotor disorder, characterized by an irresistible urge to move the legs and usually accompanied or caused by uncomfortable and unpleasant sensations)
- *Small fiber neuropathy* (small fibers are nerves found near the surface of the skin, has to do with the malfunctioning of these nerves, causing either extreme sensitivity or loss of sensation, both hot and cold), most *idiopathic* or *secondary* (primary Raynaud's phenomenon, autoimmune and Fabry' disease, our patient with *erythromelalgia*)

9.7.2
Mononeuritis Multiplex or Simplex

This is mostly seen with

- *ANCA-positive (Churg–Strauss* syndrome, *Panarteritis nodosa, Wegener's*), but also with *ANCA-negative (small vessel vasculitis,* possibly *cryoglobulinemic) vasculitis* (in an ANCA-negative female patient it began with *Mononeuritis multiplex,* then *E. coli* sepsis developed, suggesting mesenteric ischemia, with *Endocarditis verrucosa* and total destruction of all left cardiac valves)
- *RA, CTD (primary Sjögren's* syndrome) and *sarcoidosis* (facial paresis)

These two forms of neural involvement could present as a combination (*mono-/polyneuritis*) and should, particularly, in the event of *CTD* and *vasculitis,* be used as an opportunity to establish proof of a compression or *bottleneck* syndrome and involvement of the *CNS* structures.

Electromyography/nerve conduction studies and nerve/muscle biopsy (of the sural and superficial peroneal nerves) can confirm the diagnosis of the target nerve and muscles (by clinical suspicion in *PM/DM*).

9.8
Cartilage

Relapsing polychondritis (Fig. 29) is a rare but serious systemic, inflammatory rheumatic autoimmune disease, with a wide range of potential targets:

- Auricles, nasal cartilage with subsequent deformity (DD *saddle-nose* (Table 14.1) in *Wegener's*, in our case a 20-year-old woman developed for about 2 weeks without a system-/organ involvement, later associated with subacute *subglottic stenosis*), laryngeal/tracheal cartilage (*chondritides*)
- Eyes (*keratitis, epi-/scleritis, uveitis*)
- Ears (loss of hearing, vertigo, *tinnitus*)
- Joints (non-erosive *mono-/polyarthritis* → Chap. 9.3.2), as in our case (Fig. 29) in the form of *RA*-like polyarthritis
- Systemic involvement (skin → Chap. 9.1), neurological syndromes (→ Chap. 9.7), large vessels (aortitis → Chap. 9.2.2)
- Organ involvement (heart, kidneys, CNS), greater when commonly associated with other diseases (*CTD* and *vasculitis* → Part II or *myelodysplastic* syndrome)

Perhaps even more frequently, there were local forms of *auricular chondritis*, presenting with severe pain symptoms and responding surprisingly well to glucocorticoids. The systemic forms require strong immunosuppressants.

9.9
Bones or Bone Marrow

(see Chaps. 3.10 and 3.11)

- Aseptic *osteonecrosis* (Fig. 121) arises as a result of
  - *Vasculitis* (more often in *SLE*, bilateral; *giant-cell arteritis*) or in inflammatory intestinal (*Crohn's* disease) and metabolic (*diabetes mellitus*) diseases
  - Steroidal (CS 44) and immunosuppressive therapy, following radiotherapy
  - Complication of bisphosphonate therapy (affecting either the mandible or maxilla)
- Destruction of the orbita (*retrobulbar granuloma*) in *Wegener's* (Fig. 96)
- *Osteoporosis* (Chap. 3.11.1) and related *fractures*: spine (Figs. 125–127), radius, femoral neck possible:
  - *Primary* (age, estrogen deficiency, and lack of mobility)
  - *Secondary* as a result of glucocorticoid medication (CS 46), to be considered more in terms of treatment duration than dose level

- *Chronic recurrent multifocal osteomyelitis* (CRMO)/sterile osteomyelytis that commonly affects the metaphysic of long bones/associated with pustulosis palmoplantaris (Figs. 110, 111ab, 129b), pyoderma gangrenosum, severe acne, etc. (Chap. 9.1.3), and Crohn disease

Treatment is necessary when symptoms first appear (in the case of *fractures*), even as prophylaxis (in the case of risk factors or minimal *bone pain*).

System-/Organ Involvement

10

To establish the diagnosis and correctly estimate the *severity* and *prognosis* of a systemic disease, strategic and systematic screening for organ involvement should take place *upon any suspicion of such, without making any exceptions*. System-/organ involvement is always to be evaluated as an *unfavorable prognostic factor*. In contrast to connective tissue syndromes (Chap. 9), system-/organ involvement in *CTD* and/or *vasculitis* has a much broader spectrum of differential diagnosis (Chap. 14). Such systemic manifestations and broad targets, due to their unigue multifarious morphology[13,16] may change in their severity and spread over the course, or there may be a new onset, and therefore the initial clinical picture as well as that which transpires later, may be very different. In principle, *each new connective tissue and system-/organ symptom* should firstly be assigned to the *underlying disease* or its *activity* or *complications* and, if such a possibility is ruled out, consideration is given to concomitant diseases – primarily tumors (Chap. 13, Step *3*).

The *persistent and stable manifestations* of system-/organ involvement should be regarded as *irreversible damage* or the *traces* of previous activity. Hence, any organ/system involvement during chronic progression of *CTD* and/or *vasculitis* must be evaluated as a singular interaction between the *symptoms of activity* and *damage*,[5, 6, 11, 12, 19] see Chap. 13, Step *8*. The components of such a combination, which must first be explained, are to be considered as the varying targets of imminent therapy. Subsequently, only the specific and most common features of system-/organ involvement in *CTD* and *vasculitis* tend to be presented.

10.1
Kidneys (*BVAS* = maximum of *12* out of 63 points)

The *additional involvement* of the kidneys is seen in almost all patients with generalized forms of *CTD* and *vasculitis*, and in one patient even has a varied clinical pattern (from asymptomatic forms as far as irreversible and intensive care situations, e.g., *renal crisis* in *SSc* with or without hypertension, or *acute*, often rapid progressive *renal failure* in *SLE*, *SSc, microscopic polyangiitis*). The nature of the renal involvement has a tremendous influence on the *prognosis* of the diseases and often poses the main therapeutic difficulties. The kidney is often the last organ to respond to therapy.

Primary clinical and serological diagnosis should take place as early as possible, in parallel to cooperation from *nephrologists*. In comparison to *primary glomerulonephritis*, renal involvement in the case of *CTD* and *vasculitis* has more unfavorable variants – both

E. Benenson, *Rheumatology*, Symptoms and Syndromes

135

DOI: 10.1007/978-1-84996-462-3_10, © Springer-Verlag London Limited 2011

morphological (necrotizing *vasculitis*, renal infarcts) and *prognostic* (relatively rapidly developing *renal failure*, e.g., within 3 months in *rapid progressive glomerulonephritis*).

This *secondary process* should always be afforded attention in the differential diagnosis, in the case of all forms of *glomerulonephritis*. As a rule, renal biopsy is important when first establishing the diagnosis and in particular if there is *no response* to glucocorticoid therapy, in order to determine the *nature of the renal involvement* (morphological variant of *glomerulonephritis, amyloidosis, tubulointerstitial* syndrome) and follow through with the subsequent therapeutic strategy and prognosis.

Lead syndromes of renal involvement should be considered in detail at the first visit and continue to be monitored at every visit.

10.1.1
Arterial Hypertension, Malignant

Arterial hypertension stable (because of renin-mediated hypertension), possibly with crises, is highly important in

- *SSc, SLE, Microscopic polyangiitis, Panarteritis nodosa, Takayasu's arteritis* (*A. renalis* narrowing or stenosis), implying a poor prognosis, and necessitating early use of angiotensin converting enzyme (ACE) inhibitors. DD: *Fabry's* disease, *fibromuscular dysplasie.*

10.1.2
Proteinuria

(> 0.5 g/24 h or more than 3+)

- *Isolated minimal proteinuria* cannot always be treated, not even with all forms of *CTD* and *vasculitis, familial Mediterranean fever, amyloidosis, diabetic nephropathy* and e.g. *vitamin D deficiency*
- Up to 3.0 g/24 h could be proof of renal involvement in all forms of *CTD* (CS 51, 64) and *vasculitis* (CS 11) and always requires treatment. *Urinary protein diagnostics* are deduced from a 24-h urine sample (*cave*: correct collection) and comprise:
  - Protein (g/l), *proteinuria* could be *glomerular* and *tubular*
  - Albumin (g/l) suggests *selective glomerular proteinuria*
  - Electrophoresis with the question whether there is *selective* /prognostically favorable/ or *non-selective* /severe *glomerular* damage/ *proteinuria*
  - g/L crea/min
  - β2-microglobulin (*tubular* proteinuria)
- More than 3.0 g/24 h implies a *nephrotic* syndrome in two forms:
  - *Asymptomatic* (with *absence* of edema and renal insufficiency) /CS 71/ or
  - *Symptomatic* (with peripheral *edema, polyserositis*) in *glomerulonephritis, lupus nephritis* (CS 34, 38), *amyloidosis, Still's, familial Mediterranean fever, multiple myeloma, acute (Hepatitis B) und chronic liver disease*

- *Selective* minimal or moderate (<2.5 g/day) *proteinuria* (low-molecular proteins, e.g., ß2-microglobulin or alpha-1-microglobulin) is typical of *tubular* damage (CS 38 possibly due to *nephrocalcinosis* → Fig. 105)
- *Combined with hematuria* and pathological sediment (*cellular cylinders*), the disorders can be described as *glomerular.*

10.1.3
Hematuria

> 5 erythrocytes in microscopic field from midstream urine/ should be considered with the following in mind:

- *Renal hematuria* or from urinary tracts/bladder (urological consultation if necessary)
- *Renal hematuria* with *dysmorphic erythrocytes* and cellular *cylinders/casts and leukocytes* (after ruling out bacterial urinary tract infection) is a sign of *activity* (in the presence of *proteinuria*) in all forms of *CTD* and *vasculitis*
- *Micro-* or *macro*hematuria (should always be quantified over the course)
- *Isolated hematuria* possibly signifies favorable *glomerulonephritis*, generally requires no therapy (in all forms of *CTD* and *vasculitis, familial Mediterranean fever, amyloidosis*)
- *The correlation* in terms of *proteinuria* or *renal insufficiency*, whereby the most common constellations are:
  - *Massive hematuria and proteinuria* with *arterial hypertension* are signs of a *nephritic* syndrome (*SLE, Wegener's, SSc, microscopic polyangiitis*)
  - *Minimal hematuria* and *massive proteinuria* with *renal insufficiency* are signs of a *tubulointerstitial* syndrome (*SSc, drug/contrast toxicity, chronic pyelonephritis,* and amyloidosis)

10.1.4
Renal Insufficiency

Renal insufficiency is determined by the reduction in the *glomerular filtration rate* (GFR):

- Estimated or measured GFR (<50%)
- Based on *creatinine clearance* (<50 mL/min), serving as a *screening* test in early-onset *SLE*
- Based on serum *creatinine elevation* (>1.5 mg/dL).

Over the course, a distinction is made between two forms:

- ❖ *Rapid* onset and *progressive renal insufficiency* is typical of *rapid progressive glomerulonephritis*, pANCA-positive, *SLE* (CS 38), *microscopic polyangiitis, Goodpasture's* syndrome

- *Slow progressive renal insufficiency* is typical in all other forms of *CTD* and *vasculitis*, whereby a certain inefficacy (such as in refractory patients) or intolerability of the basic medication (e.g., CYC) is to be expected (CS 20, 34)
- *Unfavorable variants* of *renal insufficiency* from a clinical viewpoint are *rapid development*, elevated creatinine levels, *nephrotic* syndrome, *malignant hypertension* and (aplastic) *anemia*

10.1.5
Clinical Significance of Renal Syndromes

- *Arterial hypertension*, secondary in all forms of *CTD* and *vasculitis:*
  - *Glomerulonephritis, arteriitis* of *A. renalis* (*Takayasu's arteritis, SSc*)
    - ❖ *Prognostically unfavorable syndrome* and *most common cause of death* in *SSc, microscopic polyangiitis, Wegener's*, disease (in, *SSc* renal crisis continuous ACE inhibitor therapy required! but not the high-dose corticosteroids
  - *Secondary retinopathy* (*risk of blindness!*)
- *Nephritic* syndrome with subacute, chronic, *rapid progressive* glomerulonephritis:
  - CTD (*lupus nephritis, SSc, MCTD, PM/DM, Sjögren's* syndrome)
  - Vasculitis (*microscopic polyangiitis, Wegener's, cryoglobulinemic vasculitis* /CS 20/, *Henoch-Schönlein* purpura), rarely *Behçet's* disease or *RA*
- *Nephrotic* syndrome (membranous *lupus nephritis, secondary*/AA *amyloidosis* such as in *RA, familial Mediterranean fever,* and other *autoinflammatory* syndromes or diseases, *mixed cryoglobulinemia, Henoch-Schönlein* purpura), rare complication of NSAID, Fabry's.
- *Tubulointerstitial* syndrome (characterized by white blood cell casts in the urine sediment, with moderate proteinurie and renal insufficiency) associated with *tubulointerstitial* nephritis by *Sjögren's*, NSAIDs or allopurinol use, *sarcoidosis* (with history of nephrolithiasis), uveitis, or rarely *Behçet's* disease.
- *Renal insufficiency* (as *signs of activity* or *consequence of glomerulonephritis* – a question pivotal to *therapy and prognosis* posed at every stage of renal involvement which must be answered. To this aim the data from renal biopsy are used, enabling a prognostically important evaluation of the degree of *activity and chronification* over the course (CS 34),[3] possibly also in *Fabry's* disease.
- *Transient microhematuria* and *proteinuria* within the context of *CTD* and *vasculitis* as well as *cystitis* need to be clarified, but mostly do not require therapy.
- *Pulmonary-renal* syndrome is the clinically relevant, concurrent involvement of these organs or the acute failure (*ANCA*-associated *vasculitides*, HCV-associated *cryoglobulinemia*, and *Goodpasture's* syndrome).

10.1.6
A Lack of Renal Involvement in CTD and Vasculitis

A lack of renal involvement is quite feasible if:

- *Monosymptomatic* (with *thrombocytopenia*) *SLE* (CS 27)
- *Drug-induced and local lupus erythematosus*

- *Panarteritis nodosa* (a *discriminatory* syndrome to *microscopic polyangiitis*), though in CS 11 it is *proteinuria*
- *Churg-Strauss* syndrome /CS 72/ (rare, possibly eosinophilic interstitial nephritis)
- *Behçet's* disease (rare)

10.1.7
Genitourinary Tract Involvement

- Chronic *pyelonephritis*, recurrent under immunosuppression (CS 27)
- Chronic *cystitis* (persistent hematuria or contracted bladder in the case of *vasculitis*)
- Recurrent genital *ulcerations* (*Behçet's* disease)
- *Testicular pain* or sensitivity (*microscopic polyangiitis* /CS 12/, *Henoch-Schönlein* purpura)
- *Epididymitis* (*Behçet's* disease)
- *Orchitis* (*Wegener's* disease; *Takayasu's arteritis* in a male patient (Figs. 77ab) with acute symptoms not initially viewed as related to the underlying disease but rather as a tumor considered for orchectomy)
- *Uterus involvement* (our own observation in *Wegener's* disease)

10.2
Lungs (*BVAS* = maximum of *6* out of 63 points)

According to incidence and prognostic significance, the lungs are the second largest target for *CTD* and *vasculitis*. Any suspected primary involvement of the lungs should be investigated in light of such a fact, based on the following syndromes.

Lead symptoms: dyspnea, dry or *productive cough*, and *hemoptysis*.

10.2.1
Bronchospastic Syndrome

(FEV1 < 70%) is associated with involvement of the upper airways and bronchi, appearing as

- *Laryngitis, laryngeal edema* (in *allergy* or *hereditary angioedema*), *acute pharyngitis*/sore throat (*Still's*), *subglottic* (with stridor) or *subglottic/tracheal stenosis* (*Wegener's, histiocytosis X* /Fig. 79/). A persistent *dry cough* could be one of the first manifestations *in Sjögren's* (*bronchitis sicca*), *Still's* disease (*pharingitis*) /CS 66/ and in *giant-cell arteritis*, in one of our cases, MRI confirmed *Takayasu's arteritis* – may reflect inflammation within the arteries adjacent to cough centers – (combined with CRP elevation over 3 months) which disappeared completely after 3 days of cortisone therapy.
- ❖ *Bronchial asthma* (CS 72), also a history thereof (*Churg-Strauss* syndrome), therapy-resistant and even life-threatening *asthmatic status* could, just like *allergic rhinitis*, precede *vasculitis* for up to several years.

- *Discriminatory syndrome* for *Wegener's* disease (but not for late sequelae, Fig. 75) and *microscopic polyangiitis.*

10.2.2
Pulmonary Infiltrations, Possibly Caverns

(Clinically and radiologically, Figs. 36a, 38, 53, 75)

- *Pneumonitis* (DD in *infections, cocaine abuse*) in the form of acute onset of pulmonary insufficiency (*dyspnea, hypoxemia*), fine rales and at the same time patchy infiltrates, mostly bilateral, predominantly in the lower pulmonary lobes (Fig. 91).
- *Nodular, cavitatory* lesions, *fibrotic/shrinking* disorders of lungs (all forms of *CTD* and *vasculitis*, particularly *Wegener's* (Figs. 75, 112), *lethal midline granuloma, RA* /CS 13/, wherever tumor screening has been undertaken /Figs. 36a, 38, 39, 85/, *histiocytosis X* /Fig. 79/).
- *Pulmonary infarcts* in *pulmonary arteritis* (*giant-cell* and *Takayasu's arteritis, antiphospholipid* syndrome), alveolar (*Wegener's*) or pulmonary (*Behçet's* disease) hemorrhage.
- *Pulmonary thromboembolism* (deep venous thrombosis mostly in the lower extremities).
- *Multiple nodular foci* (relatively specific to *Wegener's*, Figs. 75, 112), also with necrosis (Fig. 112), in *rheumatoid nodules* (CS 13, Figs. 38, 39), which could cause pneumothorax (in our three cases), *Churg-Strauss* syndrome, *sarcoidosis* – predominantly hilar and/or mediastinal, stable or transitory.
- *Asymptomatic forms* of pulmonary involvement.
- Lungs involvement is not typically in classic *panarteritis nodosa*; the diagnosis of *microscopic polyangiitis* or *undifferentiated vasculitis is possible* (was in our case, the cause of death).
- Apical and elsewhere infiltrate developed in the setting of anti-TNF and in our case under MTX therapy (reactivation of tuberculosis and aspirgilosis).

10.2.3
Interstitial Fibrosis, Alveolitis, Pulmonary Arterial Hypertension (PAH)

These syndrome can develop *primary* or as a consequence of *alveolitis/ pneumonitis* (Figs. 53, 75, 91).

Clinical

- *Dyspnea* with fine rales (crepitation), mostly progressive
- Acute pulmonary decompensation with dyspnea, hypoxemia, and elevated LDH level (in immunosuppressive patients is *PCP* most likely)

- *Increased interstitial streaking* (Figs. 53, 91) in *sarcoidosis* (CS 33) often with PAH, *CTD* (CS 19) and *Wegener's* (Fig. 75), *histiocytosis X* (Fig. 79), frequently reported in *microscopic polyangiitis*
- *Diffusion* and *restrictive ventilation disorders* (*DLCO* <70% of target value), secondary criterion of *SSc* (CS 19), *MCTD* (CS 2, 30), other forms of *CTD, vasculitis* (CS 11), fibrotic *sarcoidosis, idiopathic pulmonary fibrosis*
- *Advanced fibrosis and shrinking* (*Wegener's* disease /Fig. 75/, *sarcoidosis, pneumoconiosis* in setting of the *RA* (*Caplan's* syndrome)
- *Pulmonary capillaritis* with *alveolar hemorrhage* /hemoptysis/ (*glomerulonephritis, microscopic polyangiitis, Wegener's, Churg-Srauss,* and *Goodpasture's* syndrome)
- *Pulmonary arterial hypertension* in two forms
  - *Irreversible*, more suggestive of *fibrosis* (CS 11)
  - *Unstable* during therapy, more consistent with *alveolitis* (CS 19, 30; Figs. 53, 85)

Such syndromes mostly appear with:

- *CTD* (*MCTD, SLE,* diffuse *SSc,* for *CREST* is typically the *PAH*)
- *Antisynthetase* syndrome or *anti-Jo-1* syndrome (association of *fibrosing alveolitis* and myositis-specific *anti-Jo-1* antibodies with *PM* → Chap. 11.1)
- *Vasculitis* (*Wegener's, undifferentiated vasculitis*), *sarcoidosis*
- *Idiopathic pulmonary fibrosis*/usual interstitial pneumonitis
- *RA, PsA, AS* (bilateral upper lobe fibrosis) as extraarticular symptoms
- *Seropositive RA* associated with pneumoconiosis (*Caplan's* syndrome)
- Drug-induced (MTX, Arava®, rituximab therapy)

Concomitant involvement of the lungs and kidneys is a common occurrence ("*pulmorenal* syndrome").

10.3
Heart (*BVAS* = maximum of *6* out of 63 points)

The clinically relevant, additional involvement of the heart in *CTD* and *vasculitis* is, as compared against the kidneys, more sporadic but as a rule *serious*. Accordingly, such a situation should be established quickly, as well as investigated (on first diagnosis) and treated strategically (in collaboration with cardiologists or cardiosurgeons). What is involved is *vasculitis* of the coronary vessels (*coronaritis*) within the context of *primary* systemic *vasculitis* involving the medium or large vessels (*Takayasu's* and *giant-cell arteritis, Behçet's, panarteritis nodosa, Kawasaki's* syndrome).

Even if the respective diseases are only suspected, the cardiac problems must be examined more closely. Conversely, the cardiac problems are to be initially regarded as *secondary* – particularly in patients of younger age groups – if there are no *coronary artery disease* risk factors, or if something is amiss (e. g. disproportionately high ESR

→ Chap. 8.4, CS 26). Inflammatory infestation of the small vessels and connective tissue is the reason behind the changes in the other cardiac structures.

The known *lead symptoms of cardiac involvement*, namely, *dyspnea, chest pain, cardiac arrhythmias*, could be summarized under the generic term of *cardiomyopathy*. At the same time it is wise to attempt to focus the sight on differentiated syndromes, since every syndrome or combination thereof in *CTD* and *vasculitis* could have varying diagnostic, therapeutic and prognostic outcomes. Cardiac syndromes in *CTD* and *vasculitis* are categorized as follows.

10.3.1
Coronary Syndrome

Coronary syndrome is to be viewed as a manifestation of accelerated *atherosclerosis* or *coronaritis* or *vasculopathy*, e.g., in *vasculitis* or *antiphospholipid* syndrome or in *neoplasias* → Chap. 5. It differs from the known, common diseases (*coronary heart disease, arterial hypertension*) by its clinical features, namely the lack of risk factors, possibly in young women, pain which is not always load-dependent, no clear response to nitrates, and can still be confirmed by *coronary angiogram*. Thereby, the same clinical syndromes appear:

❖ *Angina pectoris*, often *unstable* (CS 21), more in the form of *cardialgia*: completely stable, also at rest, not truly load-dependent, responding neither to nitrates nor to certain basic medications (MTX, azathioprine), but to high-dose cortisone and Arava®
❖ *Myocardial infarctions, manifest* (no difference to *coronary heart disease*) or *silent* (*SSc*)
❖ *Sudden death* by *sarcoidose* in the setting of the cardiac involvement is usually due to arrythmias
These syndromes have been seen with
  • *Vasculitis* (*Takayasu's* /CS 21/ and *giant-cell arteritis, Wegener's, panarteritis nodosa, Behçet's* /CS 26/ and *Kawasaki's*)
  • *CTD* (*SSc, SLE*, e.g., the risk of myocardial infarction in SLE women aged 35–44 years is 50-fold higher when compared with age-and sex-matched controls[20])

10.3.2
Cardiac Insufficiency and/or Cardiac Arrhythmias

Cardiac insufficiency and/or cardiac arrhythmias are *in principle* feasible in all forms of *CTD* and *vasculitis* as an expression of the *following syndromes*:

  • *Pulmonary hypertension* (*interstitial pulmonary fibrosis* in *CTD* and *vasculitis* Chap. 10.2.3) with right ventricular insufficiency
  • *Exudative pericarditis*, in the most serious cases even cardiac tamponade (*Still's, SLE, MCTD, SSc*)

- *Sicca pericarditis* is mostly only of diagnostic relevance (*SLE, RA*)
- *Myocarditis* (possible in all forms of *CTD, Still's, Takayasu arteritis*)
- *Endocarditis* or *valvular involvement*
  - A diastolic or systolic sound > 3/6 is of relevance
  - In *SLE* (Libman-Sacks verrucous endocarditis), *valvular involvement* in *antiphospholipid* syndrome, *Takayasu's arteritis, Churg-Strauss* syndrome, *sepsis* (*B. coli sepsis* with massive destruction to all left cardiac valves, requiring surgery, was an acute development in a male patient with ANCA-negative *vasculitis*, probably due to mesenteric ischemia)
- *Myocardial fibrosis (cardiomyopathy), diffuse* and also *focal* (*SSc*) with diastolic dysfunction and high incidence of conduction disturbance (also because of the fibrosis of the conducting tissue)
- *Cardiomyopathy*, cardiac involvement with no further differentiation, or *Fabry's* disease, involving echocardiographic detection of ventricular dysfunction
- *Arrhythmias* as signs of these diseases; may result from the effects of drugs (such as hydroxychloroquine) or antibodies (e.g., *anti-SS-Ro*-Ab)

Such syndromes often determine the *prognosis* and *cause of death* (e.g., in *SLE, SSc* the most common cause of death is accelerated *atherosclerosis*), should be established as early on as possible, linked to the lead symptoms and controlled actively by collaborating with a cardiologist.

10.4
Serosa

The involvement of all three types of serosa (*polyserositis*) is in fact an uncommon, but relatively specific phenomenon in *CTD*, especially *SLE* (elevated ANA and dsDNA antibodies could be found in the punctate), *MCTD, Sjögren's* syndrome, *rheumatic fever, Still's, JIA, RA, familial Mediterranean fever* and certain forms of *vasculitis* (*Wegener's*), but also their complications (e.g., intestinal perforation in *cANCA*-positive vasculitis, CS 48) and potentially concomitant diseases (*pneumonia, TB, sepsis*), which could develop as a *primary* spontaneous *or secondary* phenomenon under immunosuppression.

10.4.1
Pericarditis

Pericarditis is to be interpreted as a sign of the *cardiac involvement* of a systemic disease, but has a broad spectrum of differential diagnosis (cardiological aspects, amyloidosis, and tumors):

- *Pericarditis exsudativa* is viewed as a *sign of activity*, mostly in *SLE* (10–30%), *SSc* (often related to pulmonary arterial hypertension), *Still's* and *RA* with potentially minimal *arthralgias*, presenting in the form of

- *Pericardial pain, dyspnea and percardial effusion*
  - ❖ *Cardiac tamponade* (in severe cases) is to be suspected in the case of
    - Massive *dyspnea*
    - Pronounced retrolingual and *jugular* veins (on inspection)
    - Weakened, soft cardiac tones
    - *Low cardiac output* syndrome (tachycardia, hypotension, elevated central venous pressure, possibly *cardiac arrest*)
    - *Hepatomegaly* and *legs edema*
- *Pericarditis sicca* is mostly a sign of previous *pericarditis exsudativa* in the aforementioned diseases and should be viewed more retrospectively. It presents as
  - *Pericardial pain, rub*
  - *Adhesions* on imaging (ECG, echocardiogram and chest X-ray)

10.4.2
Pleuritis

Pleuritis appears within the context of multiorgan involvement in all forms of *CTD* and *vasculitis*, or could be monosymptomatic or combined with *arthritis* (variant of chronic *SLE*).

Clinical

- *Pleuritis exsudativa* is an indicator of *active* systemic disease, characterized by
  - *Dyspnea* and restrictive *pulmonary insufficiency* (the initial symptoms in one patient with *SSc*, CS 19; in one female patient with seropositive, active *RA*, *exudative pleuritis* was not viewed within the context of *RA*, but as "unknown etiology")
  - Weakened percussion, diminished respiratory sounds in the lower lobes
  - Typical radiological finding In diagnostic and therapeutic terms, it is essential to perform *pleural puncture* to examine the pleural fluid and resolve the following question:
  - *Exudate* or *transudate*
  - Degree of *activity*, e.g., from *CRP* elevation, and
  - *Disease specificity* (*ANA, RF, tumor* cells)
- *Pleuritis sicca* and *pleural fibrosis* are to be viewed as the result of inflammation and appear in all forms of *CTD* and *vasculitis, familial Mediterranean fever* (diagnostic criterion) as
  - *Shortness of breath* due to pleuritic pain with
  - *Pleural rub and pleural thickening*
  - *Restricted mobility* of the diaphragm (clinically and radiologically)

10.4.3
Peritonitis

Peritonitis or even a suspicion thereof (Chap. 10.5.6) is to be treated as a *life-threatening condition* (in some forms of *CTD* and *vasculitis*). Differentiation should be made between:

- *Peritonial irritation* (peritonism), an *irritable condition* of the peritoneum, e.g., in *Henoch -Schönlein* purpura, *rheumatic fever, arteriitis* of the abdominal vessels as part of *familial Mediterranean fever* (diagnostic criterion), *Takayasu's ateritis, Still's* and *Behçet's* diseases
- ❖ *Peritonitis* is an *acute abdominal condition,* seen in particular with *ANCA-positive* necrotizing *vasculitis (Wegener's, Panarteritis nodosa)* in the following forms:
  - *Intestinal perforations* due to *mesenteric thrombosis* /CS 48/
  - *Massive gastrointestinal hemorrhage* (also drug-induced, *NSAID*)
  - *Thrombosis, renal* (CS 29) and *mesenteric (atherosclerosis),* and *thromboembolism (antiphospholipid* syndrome, *Behçet's*)

These patients are to be treated cooperatively and *as early as possible* by a surgeon.

10.5
Gastrointestinal Tract (*BVAS* = maximum of *6* out of 63 points)

Gastroenterological syndromes have developed relatively frequently, in varied forms, with *CTD* and *vasculitis* and/or as a side effect to ongoing therapy (e. g. *gastritis* as response to many DMARDs and NSAIDs and particularly associated with RA and other rheumatic diseases). *Lead symptoms* and *syndromes: dysphagia, swallowing disorders, abdominal pain, Angina abdominalis,* and *diarrhea* with or without *bleeding, weight loss, positive hepatitis B* and *C.*

10.5.1
Diarrhea

- *Reactive arthritis* (yersiniosis; Campylobacter enteritis; salmonellosis)
- *CTD* (intestinal infestation)
- *Vasculitis* (intestinal and vascular infestation)
- *Arthropathy (Crohn's, Colitis ulcerosa)*
- *During immunosuppression* (opportunistic infections; common with Arava®)
- *Fabry's* disease (combined with *malabsorption,* abdominal cramps).

10.5.2
Dysphagia and Swallowing Disorders

- *Motility disorders of the esophagus* (*esophageal rigidity*; secondary *achalasia, esophageal hypomobility*), and/or profound *gastrointestinal hypomotility* in *SSc* (CS 19), *CREST* (CS 58), *MCTD* (CS 24)
- *Esophagitis*
- *Fibromyalgia* (with glomus sensation)
- *Hypomobility* of the head joints (C0/C1/C2 blockade in the region of Fig. 60)
- *Abdominal motility disorders* in the form of *reflux esophagitis* (heartburn).

10.5.3
Malabsorption

Malabsorption suggests intestinal or gastrointestinal involvement linked to a poor prognosis (*Panarteriitis nodosa* /CS 48/, *SSc, CREST* syndrome, *Behçet's*).

10.5.4
Hepatolienal Syndrome

Hepatolienal syndrome should be regarded (provided other diseases have been ruled out) as an *infestation of the liver* or the *reticuloendothelial system*, or *hemolysis*, in all forms of *CTD* and *vasculitis,* and *JIA*

- *Hepatomegaly*
    - *Primary biliary cirrhosis* and *autoimmune cholangitis* (*SSc* and *CREST* syndrome)
    - *Hepatitis* in *SLE, MCTD, Still's*
    - *Lupoid hepatitis* and *autoimmune hepatitis* (*ANA*-positive)
    - *Granulomatous inflammation* (*sarcoidosis,* among others)
    - Fatty liver (*drug toxicity, diabetes mellitus*)
    - *Vasculitis* (*cryoglobulinemic*) in *hepatitis C* (CS 20)
    - *Gaucher's* (with splenomegaly)
- *Splenomegaly* associated with
    - *Leukocytopenia* and *lymphadenopathy* (*Felty's* syndrome, CS 68)
    - *Hemolytic anemia* (may be a form of *SLE*)
    - *Vasculitis* (*cryoglobulinemic*)
- *Hepatorenal* syndrome is the clinically relevant, concurrent involvement of these organs or the acute failure of both.

10.5.5
Elevated Liver Enzymes

(*GOT* and/or *GPT* or *GGT*) in

- *CTD* (*Sjögren's* syndrome, *SLE, SSc, PM/DM*)
- *Still's* (CS 62, often with *LDH*)
- *Vasculitis* (*Panarteritis nodosa, cryoglobulinemic*, CS 20)
- *Autoimmune hepatitis*
- Drug-induced (MTX, CYC, Arava®, Enbrel®, etc).

10.5.6
Abdominal Pain

- *Subacute, chronic peritonitis* (CS 48) or *peritonial irritation, perihepatitis, perisplenitis*
- *Angina abdominalis* (*Henoch-Schönlein* purpura, *panarteritis nodosa, atherosclerosis*)
- *Colic-type* (*cryoglobulinemic* vasculitis /CS 20/, *Henoch-Schönlein* purpura, *lupus enteritis, Fabry's, acute porphyria*)
- *With episodes of fever*, recurrent (*familial Mediterranean fever*)
- *Ileus* and *mesenteric infarctions* (in *vasculitis* /CS 48/, *CTD* /CS 29/)
- *Pancreatitis* (*vasculitis, SLE, Sjögren's, „autoimmune pancreatitis"* in the setting of *IgG4*-related systemic disease associated with lymphoplasmatic infiltration into a variety of organs /aorta, salivary glands, kidney, and others organs[23])
- *Inflammatory bowel disease* (*Crohn's*, Colitis ulcerosa)
- Aortitis (Fig. 77), Arteritis mesenterica in *Takayasu's arteritis* (cortisone-dependent pain)
- *Angioedema, hereditary* (recurrent, possibly with symptoms of *ileus*)
- *Diverticulitis* (also back pain, fever, peritonial irritation, perforation)

10.6
Central Nervous System (*BVAS* = maximum of *9* out of 63 points)

The case here is primarily *CNS* vasculitis (synonym: *primary angiitis of the CNS* /PACNS/), in fact the involvement potentially of all structures. Combined with the involvement of the peripheral nervous system (Chap. 9.7) the neurological symptoms as a whole represent one of the most common of all forms of *CTD* (excepting *SSc* in the sense of organ involvement; the damage may occur as a result of arterial hypertension) and *vasculitis*.

Lead symptoms and syndromes of *CNS vasculitis* may cover the entire spectrum of neurology and psychiatry, namely subacute development of *headache, convulsions, psychoses, numbness, sensory and motor disorders in the extremities, mood disorders, cognitive impairment, impaired vision, cerebral conduction disorders,* positive /*white metallic*/ *MRI* finding (Fig. 50), *seizure,* or *multifocal strokes* with *infarction* syndrome (Fig. 17), or chronic *meningitis.*

Some neurological syndromes could be *drug-induced,* such as in one tragic case I have experienced: a 16-year-old girl with an episode of *SLE* (crisis) developed irreversible *cerebral edema* with *fatal outcome* following intra-venous glucocorticoid infusion. There have been recent reports of progressive multifocal *leukoencephalopathy (PML)* under treatment with certain medications (CellCept®, rituximab). But most often our patients with neurological symptoms are suffering from *CNS vasculitis.* A differentiation is made between *two forms* and several clinical *syndromes.*

10.6.1
Forms of CNS Vasculitis

- *Primary* isolated *CNS* /PACNS/, characterized by vasculitis limited to brain and spinal cord, presents in a subacute manner with slowly evolving encephalopathy, and multifocal strokes. The definitive diagnosis requires an angiogram of intracranial arteries (showing segmental narrowing), MRI, CSF analysis or brain biopsy
- *Secondary CNS* involvement as a result of
  - *Primary* (CS 6) *and secondary APS* (Chap. 11.4) or, e.g., in *RA* (female patient with secondary *vasculitis* /Fig. 100/ and use of Vioxx® /during the period in which it was approved/ developed transient *CNS* symptoms potentially attributable to both causes)
  - *SLE* and other forms of *CTD* (*juvenile Sjögren's* syndrome, CS 18)
  - *Secondary vasculitis* or *vasculopathies*
    - *Atherosclerosis,* vasospasm associated with hypertension or hemorrhage
    - *Sarcoidosis* (CNS involvement can exist without active pulmonary disease)
    - *Infections, sepsis, lymphoproliferative* diseases, *lethal midline granuloma, drugs* (e.g., cocaine, allopurinol)
  - *Primary systemic vasculitis* (in approx. 5–50%)
    - *Giant-cell arteritis* (if possible quickly prescribe corticoids), *panarteritis nodosa, Wegener's, Takayasu's arteritis, Behçet's*
  - *Neuropathic Gaucher's* (non-inflammatory storage disease)
  - *Acute intermittent porphyria*
  - Beriberi (Vitamin B deficiency)
  - *Reversible cerebral vasoconstriction* syndrome (Chap. 8.3) with the onset of a thunderclap headache, include the different conditions, such as migraine, hypertensive encephalopathy, postpartum state, and exposure to vasoconstrictive drugs

10.6.2
Clinical Syndromes

- *Encephalopathy:*
  - *Meningoencephalitis*
  - *Aseptic meningitis* (in *primary CNS* vasculitis)
  - *Diffuse encephalopathy* with impairment of cognitive functions
  - *Focal* cerebral involvement with *apoplectic insults, hemiparesis,* transitory ischemic attacks in *SLE, Sjögren's* syndrome (CS 18), *antiphospholipid* syndrome (CS 6), *vasculitis, Fabry's* disease
  - *Epilepsy* (seizures could be monosymptomatic, variant of chronic *SLE, Chorea minor* /CS 71/ also a primary criterion of *rheumatic fever*)
- *Cranial nerve neuritis* (myosis, ptosis, numbness in the cheeks) in *giant-cell arteritis, polymyalgia rheumatica*
  - Cranial nerve II: visual disorders (as far as *blinding*)
  - Cranial nerve VIII: attacks of dizziness, *tinnitus, impaired hearing*
- *Myelitis* (spinal involvement) with symptoms of *paraplegia* (CS 18 and 64), as in compression fracture (CS 46)
  - Weakness or sensory losses in the lower extremities
  - Loss of control of the sphincter (rectum and bladder)

10.6.3
No CNS Involvement

This is the case, as a rule, in
- *Drug-induced SLE*
- *SSc* (except for complications caused by *arterial hypertension*)

10.7
Exocrine Glands

Most often, *autoimmune exocrinopathy* is involved, taking the form of inflamed salivary, tear and other exocrine glands (*sicca syndrome of mucosal surface*), presenting *clinically, immunologically, and histologic* as *primary Sjögren's* syndrome or disease, or *secondary Sjögren's* syndrome (with other diseases). In the case of *primary Sjögren's* syndrome, an increased rate of *lymphoma* (Chap. 5) should always be kept in mind.

The sicca symptoms far exceed the *Sjögren's* syndrome and could arise from other, non-immunological causes.

**10.7.1
Sicca Syndrome**

Affecting, above all:

- Mouth (*xerostomia, xeilitis*): persistent (>3 months) daily dry mouth and frequent consumption of drinks to aid swallowing of dry foods, salivary flow measurement and parotid scintigraphy)
- Eyes (*xerophthalmia, xerokeratitis*): deficient lacrimation in Schirmer test, recurrent sand grain sensation (>3 months) and use of artificial tear fluid, conjunctival injection such a rose bengal staining, possibly corneal defects
- Bronchial dryness is a predilection to develop inspissated mucus plugs and a chronic, non-productive cough (bronchitis sicca)
- Skin (desquamation) and vagina (*thrush*).

When examining the sicca symptoms, consideration should be given to *three conditions*:

- *Primary Sjögren's* syndrome, as the most common autoimmune disease of all, has specific *histologic* (focal lymphocytic infiltration of the exocrine glands, determined by a biopsy of the minor labial salivary glands), *immunological* (Chap. 11.1) and *clinical constellations*:
  - *Arthralgias, myalgias, lymphadenopathy* (CS 49), *neuropathies* (CS 18)
  - *Vasculitis (purpura /CS 56/ as in Figs. 56ab), Raynaud's* syndrome
  - *Pulmonary involvement (fibrosis, pneumonitis, pleuritis /CS 49/)*
  - *Tubulointerstitial renal damage* with *nephrocalcinosis* (as in Fig. 105), *glomerulonephritis*
  - *Gastrointestinal tract (gastritis, pancreatitis, primary biliary cirrhosis)*
  - *Lupus* type *skin changes* (CS 49), *myopathy* and possibly transformation into a *lymphoma* (CS 56) → Chap. 5.

The progression of *primary Sjögren's* syndrome is mostly relatively favorable in clinical terms, with isolated sicca symptoms which relatively seldom require systemic immunosuppressive therapy (only local replacement therapy).

In isolated cases, however, this disease has been of an *extremely dramatic, even urgent nature*, such as in a 13-year-old girl (CS 18) with recurrent neurological and *visual deficits* which, over the course of 3 years, were interpreted as *MS* and treated as such, or in a 65-year-old woman (CS 56) in whom, over an observation period of 12 years, two forms of *lymphoma* and a thus related *emergency* situation developed; or in a 40-year-old woman (CS 48) in whom the disease presented with acute *exudative pleuritis* and *lymphadenopathy*.

- *Secondary Sjögren's* syndrome is a concomitant symptom with:
  - *RA,* all forms of *CTD* (almost always in *SSc, CREST* syndrome /CS 32/, *MCTD*)

- *Impaired esophageal motility* (in this, and other diseases)
- Chronic *Hepatitis C, HIV* infection
- *Sarcoidosis*
- *Amyloidosis*
- *Lipoproteinemias* type IV and V
- *Still's* disease
- *Hyperthyroidism*, autoimmune thyroiditis, diabetes mellitus
- Negative testing for antibodies to the *Ro/SS-A* and *La/SS-B*

For *Sjögren's* syndrome to be diagnosed, the symptoms must persist for *at least 3 months*.

- *Non-autoimmune conditions* with *sicca* symptoms differ in their timing and their etiology:
  - Medications (beta-blockers, antidepressants, antihistamines, MTX, diuretics, antihypertensive)
  - Wearers of contact lenses
  - Psychogenic
  - Irradiation
  - *Infections*, acute and chronic (e.g., pharyngitis).

10.7.2
Parotid Enlargement

Parotid enlargement can be established clinically, by ultrasound and scintigram. On seeing a "*fat cheek*," thoughts should turn to:

- *Sjögren's* syndrome (CS 56, whereby the increased mass was the initial sign of *lymphoma*)
- *Wegener's*
- *Heerfordt's* syndrome (including fever, uveitis, facial paresis, arthralgias in *sarcoidosis*)
- Lymphoma (*bihilar lymphadenopathy* is typical of *sarcoidosis*, Fig. 91)
- Bacterial, *viral and calcified parotid* (mumps, influenza, HIV, cytomegalovirus, and Coxsackie; *secondary* infection, chronic sclerosing sialadenitis)
- Endocrine (sialadenosis associated with diabetes mellitus, acromegaly)

In the event of *unilateral enlargement, neoplasias*, bacterial *infection*, and chronic *sialodenitis* can be expected. If the *involvement* is *bilateral, viral* (mumps, influenza, Epstein-Barr virus, cytomegalovirus, HIV) and *granulomatous diseases* (*sarcoidosis, Wegener's, TB*) are possible.

10.8
Eyes (*BVAS* for eyes and mucosa = maximum of *6* out of 63 points)

Ocular involvement in its myriad forms is one of the most common associations in rheumatology patients. *Lead symptoms and syndromes: pain, "red eyes," impaired visions, exophtalmus*, whether transient, the just as important anamnestic evidence, or the consequence of ophthalmologically prescribed cortisone therapy. If such problems arise, *ophthalmological consultation* should be arranged. Such an approach has been taken on board with greater success by ophthalmologists, I believe, since today almost every patient with inflammatory ocular symptoms is referred for rheumatological consultation.

This was the case in one female, 60-year-old patient with the clinical diagnosis of *polymyalgia rheumatica*. The progression of the disease was fairly untypical on account of being rather young and responding poorly to cortisone, with increasing B symptoms. In excess of the standard procedures (her husband was an oncologist), *tumor screening* was performed but revealed no findings. As the vision deteriorated an ophthalmological consultation took place. Quite surprisingly, screening for *breast carcinoma* was advised, whereupon an *intraductal tumor* was in fact identified, in an already advanced stage.

At the end of the day it is important to understand that *any ocular structure*, and even the *periorbita*, may be affected by our (and oncological) diseases. Moreover, the *impact of cortisone therapy* (e.g., cataracts) and increased intraocular pressure (*secondary glaucoma*) must be kept in mind.

10.8.1
Conjunctivitis, Scleritis, Keratitis

Multiple causes can involve the external ocular structure mostly in association with systemic symptoms includes a broad variety of autoimmune and idiopathic inflammatory conditions, and infections.

- *Episcleritis* (painless "red eyes" with vague discomfort does not pose a risk to vision)
  - *Wegener's*
  - *RA*
  - *PsA*
  - *Inflammatory bowel disease*
- *Scleritis* (Fig. 57, painful "red eyes" often in comparison with impaired visions, *episcleritis* or corneal ulceration in the setting of the systemic disease)
  - *Rheumatoid vasculitis*
  - *SpA*
  - *Wegener's* (as well *conjunctivitis* and *episcleritis*)
  - *Scleritis* can cause such complications as *uveitis*, or *optic neuropathy*
- *Keratitis* in some case with corneal ulceration (peripheral ulcerative keratitis-PUK), and is potential consequence, corneal melt in setting of patients with

- *RA*
- *Wegener's*
- *AS* and *Sjögren's* (own cases: PUK with transplantation of the cornea)
- *SSc*
- *Cogan's* syndrome associated with audiovestibular dysfunction and large-medium vessel vasculitis
- *Fabry's* disease (deposits in the *cornea*).

10.8.2
Uveitis (Iritis, Iridocyclitis)

These disorders associated often with

- HLA-B27 in *AS* (strong association), *ReA, PsA*, or *inflammatory bowel disease* and cause a highly symptomatic *anterior uveitis* (synonyms iritis) most unilateral, and self-limited within several months
- Unlike the *RA* and *Wegener's*, it is usually *(epi)-scleritis* and ulcerative *keratitis*
- *Posterior uveitis* (toxoplasmose, in *Behçet's* is associated with *hypopyon*)
- *Uveitis* is common also in the setting of a
  - *Wegener's*
  - *JIA* (associated with inflammatory exudates overling the peripheral retina the most common form of *uveitis* in childhood)
  - *Sarcoidosis* in the form of the *Heerfordt's* (a combination with the inflammation of the lacrimal and parotis glands, and cranial neuropathy) and *Löfgren's* syndrome (a combination with the erythema nodosum and polyarthritis)
  - *Cogan's*
  - Tubulointerstitial *nephritis* /TINU/ is associated with fever and arthralgies
  - *MS* (associated with optic neuritis and peripheral retinal periphlebitis)
  - *Infections* (e.g., syphilis)
  - *Drugs* (e.g., biphosphonates, any antibiotics)
  - Many cases of uveitis (up to 50%) remain *idiopathic*

10.8.3
Retinopathies

Possibly with *retinal exudation* or *hemorrhaging* or *retinal artery occlusion* are seen commonly in patients with

- SLE
- Vasculitides /retinal involvement in Wegener's is relatively uncommon)

- APS
- Behçet's disease
- Hypertension
- HIV
- Seldom in borreliosis
- Septic emboli secondary to subacute or lenta bacterial endocarditis
- *Hydroxychloroquine* therapy, dose dependent
- Metastasis as indicated above for mamma carcinoma.

Possible with *proiferative and hypertensive* changes are seen commonly in patients with

- *Takayasu arteritis* (in the setting of renal artery stenosis)
- *Infections* (toxoplasmosis) often in setting of immunosuppression (herpes simplex, herpes zoster, or cytomegalovirus)

10.8.4
Optic Neuritis or Neuropathy

With visual affectation, such as in *Sjögren's* syndrome with *CNS vasculitis* (CS 18) or *optical atrophy, double vision* (diplopia) or *cranial nerve neuritis II* (*polymyalgia rheumatica, giant-cell arteritis, MS, sarcoidosis, Behçet's,* and *borreliosis*).

10.8.5
Periorbital Processes

Cortisone-dependent *ocular pain, orbital granuloma* or *pseudotumor* with destruction of the orbital wall are seen commonly in patients with

- Wegener's /Fig. 96/
- Sarcoidosis
- Lethal midline granuloma
- Cogan's
- Lymphomas
- Eye muscle myositis
- Exophthalmus is associated with
  - Histiocytosis X, see comments on Fig. 79
  - Hyperthyroidism
  - Orbital granuloma
  - Sarcoidosis

10.8.6
Strabism

Crossed eyes or lack of motor coordination in both eyes are seen commonly in patients with in *PM/DM*.

10.8.7
Amaurosis Fugax

Amaurosis fugax and visual loss (CS 18) or visual field defects

- Involvement of the *A. ophtalmica* in *giant-cell arteritis, polymyalgia rheumatica* (corticoids *before confirming diagnosis!*), *Behçet's* (the most common cause of *blindness* in Japan)
- Vitreous bleeding, possibly leading to sudden *blindness* or *deteriorated vision* (*SpA, giant-cell arteritis*)

10.8.8
Eye Muscle Involvement

Eye muscle involvement was assumed in a 38-year old female: *orbital pain, dose-dependent, prompt response to corticoids, CK-MB* elevation up to 60% with no increase in CK or troponin in the serum and no cardiac symptoms.

10.8.9
Cataract

(Lense opacity) are seen commonly in patients under cortisone therapy.

10.9
ENT (*BVAS* = maximum of 6 out of 63 points)

Such problems are seen just as often and very dramatically (see below) as ocular symptoms, particularly in the case of *vasculitis*, requiring the relevant symptoms to be examined by a specialist as early as possible.

Lead symptoms are *nasal congestion* with *scab formation/polyposis* and *bleeding, hoarseness, earache, dizziness, deafness, non-productive cough, dyspnea.* Syndromes arising as a result may be attributed to the following structures:

10.9.1
Throat

- Recurrent *pharyngitis* (associated with active *Still's* disease)
- ❖ *Subglottic stenosis* (*Wegener's*)
- *Laryngitis* (if *hoarseness* lasts more than 3 weeks, it should be investigated rheumatologically to rule out hypo-hyperthyroidism /*SSc, MCTD, vasculitis, polyneuropathies/*)
- *Laryngeal neuropathy* (associated with mononeuritis in *SLE*, and small vessel vasculitis)

10.9.2
Nose

- Granulomatous inflammations of the maxillary sinuses (Fig. 86) possibly orbita, resistant to therapy (*Wegener's*)
- Nasal septal perforation (*Wegener's, MCTD, relapsing polychondritis, sarcoidosis*)
- Allergic or hemorrhagic *rhinitis* with ulcerations (also painless) and tissue destruction of the midface, typical of *Wegener's* (Fig. 96), *Churg-Strauss* syndrome (could precede vasculitis by a number of years), *lethal midline granuloma*
- Possibly *aseptic necrosis* in the maxillary region during biphosphonate therapy

It is *essential* to diagnosis, ultimately, to *biopsy* the *ENT* region.

10.9.3
Ears

The above-mentioned ocular findings often go together with audivestibular symptoms, and do not always simultaneously with system-/organ involvement.

- *Otitis media* with aural discharge (*Wegener's*)
- Cochlear or audiovestibular dysfunction with vertigo and tinntus as
  - A part of immune-mediated inner ear disease (IMIED) in association with such autoimmune condition as *Sjögren', Wegener's, Cogan's* or *giant-cell arteritis,*
  - As signs of the *Meniere's* disease has many years of history (unlike short-term history of IMIED)
  - In association with drugs (aminoglucosides, antimalarials, NSAIDs)
  - Sarcoidosis

- Infection (secondary and tertiary syphilis)
- Possibly affecting the nose in the setting of the *relapsing polychondritis* (Fig. 29)
- As isolated entity.
- *Deafness*
  - *Wegener's,* and *sarcoidosis*
  - *Cogan's* syndrome, associated with interstitial *keratitis, vasculitis* in form of aortitis, renal artery stenosis, or occlusion of the great vessels
  - *Sudden autoimmune sensorineural hearing loss* – as other part of immune-mediated inner ear disease (IMIED), cortisone-dependent audiovestibular dysfunction, *primary or secondary,* e. g. associated with *CNS* vasculitis /CS 6/), other *vasculitides* (Wegener's, polyarteritis nodosa, giant cell arteritis), and *Sjögren*'s
- Autoinflammatory diseases
  - *Muckle-Wells* syndrome is dominantly inherited disease characterized by sensorineural deafness in association with rashes, fever, arthralgia, high serum level of *CRP,* and e. g. amyloidosis A; the recovery following anakinra treatment, IL-1-receptor antagonist, see Chap. 7.3.2, 8.1 is described
  - *Periodic fever syndrome, Still's* disease (responsible to IL-1-antibody, Canakinumab® → Chap. 7.3.2, 8.1), already permissed for these diseases
  - Familial Mediterranean Fever
- Atypical manifestation by *giant-cell arteritis* in our series cases. Thus was interpreted the following relations: 65 old man, acute symmetric *deafness* with headache and *hight level of CRP* (up to factor *x 64),* inconspicuous both the *MRI* of the brain and antibody spectrum, complete regression of the headache and CRP from puls-glucocorticods (was made before the biopsy of *a. temporalis*) without influence on the *deafness* (like the ears involvement in the outcomes by this illness).

10.10
Blood and Reticuloendothelial System

These systems are almost always affected by rheumatic diseases, initially and monosymptomatically in

- *Hemolysis* or *thrombocytopenic purpura* (Fig. 78), in *SLE* (CS 27, 51, 64)
- *Lymphadenopathy* in *Still's* (CS 66) or *Sjögren's* syndrome (CS 49) or *lymphoma* (CS 59), *Felty's* syndrome (CS 68)
- Various diseases, potentially with *complications* and ongoing therapy
  Such changes should be viewed relatively broadly, with possible consideration of
- *Disease-specific* syndromes (e.g., isolated *leukopenia* in *Felty's* syndrome or *hemolysis* or *thrombocytopenia* in *SLE*)
- *Activity parameters* (possibly in all inflammatory rheumatic diseases, as a distinction to non-inflammatory diseases)
- *Complications* (bleeding, sepsis and other infections)
- *Signs of an effect* (cytostatics) *and adverse effects* (gastric bleeding)
- *Criteria* for an exclusion diagnosis of *hematological disease* (e.g., *lymphoma* in *RA* and *Sjögren's* syndrome) or *paraneoplasia* (Chap. 5)

10.10.1
Anemia

(Hb <10 g/dL)

- Normochromic (*seldom* <9 g/dl)

Blood count

- Normocytic
- Serum iron decreased
- Ferritin often increased

Clinical

- *Activity parameters* in chronic inflammatory diseases,
  - Often in *RA, polymyalgia rheumatica, panarteritis nodosa, Takayasu's arteritis*
  - *Renal insufficiency* (*CTD* and *vasculitis*), unfavorable prognosis
- Hypochromic (*often* <9 g/dl)

Blood count

- Microcytic
- Serum iron decreased
- Ferritin decreased or normal

Clinical

- *Gastrointestinal bleeding* often under
  - NSAIDs and corticoids
  - Basic therapeutics: sulfasalazine, cytostatics
- Hemolytic

Blood count

- Reticulocytosis
- Fragmentocytes
- Haptoglobin
- Bilirubin indirect

- LDH
- *Coombs* test positive

Clinical

- *CTD*, could be monosymptomatic in chronic *SLE*
- *Vasculitis, familial Mediterranean fever, Felty's* syndrome
- ❖ *Moschcowitz* syndrome, *primary or secondary,* e.g., in *SLE* (CS 64):
  - Association with hemolytic microangiopathy and fragmentocytosis
  - Thrombocytopenia
  - Acute renal failure, neurological deficits

10.10.2
Thrombocytopenia and Thrombocytosis

(<100,000/µL and >450,000/µL, respectively)

- *Thrombocytopenia*
  - *Autoimmune / immunological*
    - In *CTD* and *vasculitis, antiphospholipid* syndrome (Chap. 11.4), *Felty's* syndrome (CS 68)
    - Could be *monosymptomatic* (in *SLE*, CS 27)
  - *Drug-induced and toxic* (DMARD's, NSAID's, gold)
    - Heparin-induced
  - *Genetical* (*Wiskott-Aldrich* syndrome is an X-linked recessive disorder characterized by thrombocytopenia, bleeding, small platelets, eczema, recurrent infections, IgA-nephritis and immunodeficiency).
- *Thrombocytosis* can be seen with
  - Highly active, inflammatory rheumatic diseases (*vasculitis,* e.g., *TA*)
  - Acute bleeding
  - Iron deficiency
  - Essential (thrombocytemia).

10.10.3
Leukopenia and Leukocytosis

(Less than 4,000/µL and >10,000/µL, respectively)

- *Leukopenia* (principally *neutropenia*):
  - *Autoimmune / immunological*
    - *Felty's* syndrome (neutrophil count<2000/µL for at least 6 months) combined with *arthritis* and *splenomegaly*, CS 68)

- *LGL* ("*large granular lymphocyte* syndrome") is a *lymphoproliferative* syndrome (*T-cell* leukemia) associated with *RA, Felty's* and *Sjögren's* syndrome
- *Active SLE*, selective (< 3000/µL leukocytes) or combined with other forms of *cytopenia*
- *Sjögren's* syndrome (associated with recurrent infection, and thrombocytopenia)
- Not usually associated with *primary vasculitis* (also applies to thrombocytopenia)
- *Drug toxicity* (basic therapeutics, particularly MTX, NSAID's)
- *Leukocytosis* (mostly belongs to acute-phase reaction)
  - *Autoimmune / immunological*
    - *Systemic vasculitis*
    - *Still's, RA* (acute episodes)
  - *Medicinal*
    - Corticoids
    - *Infections*
- *Eosinophilia* (*absolute* increase > 500/µL in the blood)
  - *Churg-Strauss* syndrome (more than 10% in the blood combined with *bronchial asthma, polyneuropathies*, CS 72; *panarteritis nodosa*, CS 48)
  - *Sjögren's* syndrome
  - *Löffler* syndrome
  - Eosinophilic *fasciitis* (Chap. 9.4.4)
  - *Hypereosinophil* syndrome (feverish episodes, chronic respiratory tract infections, chronic *eosinophilic pneumonia*)
  - *Eosinophilic myalgia* syndrome
  - *Allergy* or *bronchial asthma*
  - *Parasitic infection*
  - *Eosinophilic leukemia*
- Acquired *hemophilia* (clinical: *bleeding*, immunological: *factor VIII* antibodies) in *CTD, Behçet's, infections, lymphomas.*

10.10.4
Hemoglobinopathy

Hemoglobinopathy in the form of

- *Hemochromatosis* (CS 50)
- *Thalassemia*
- *Sickle-cell anemia*

10.10.5
Reticuloendothelial Syndrome

- *Lymphadenopathy* is characterized by lymph node /*axillary, mandibular, hilar* (Fig. 91), *inguinal* / enlargement, which should be established by clinical and radiological examination (ultrasound, X-ray, chest and abdominal CT).

  Such a syndrome, which when pronounced is described as *pseudolymphoma*, is part of the clinical pattern of
  - *CTD* (*SLE, Sjögren's* syndrome /CS 49/, *MCTD*) when generalized
  - *Still's* disease (CS 66)
  - *Sarcoidosis* (CS 33)
  - *Lymphoproliferative* diseases (CS 59), the incidence of which is increased with *RA* and *Sjögren's* syndrome (Chap. 5)
  - *Churg-Strauss* syndrome (the difference from the other vasculitides).
- *Hepatomegaly* and/or *splenomegaly* (Chap. 10.5.4)
  - In all forms of *CTD* and *vasculitis*
  - *Arthropathies* (*hemochromatosis*)
  - *HIV, Still's, sarcoidosis*
  - Opportunistic *infections* (under immunosuppression)
- *Macrophage activation* (*MAS*) or *hemophagocytic* syndrome occurs in patients with autoimmune diseases or *lymphoma* (rarely in primarily healthy subjects); its nosological classification is unclear. The triggers may be infections or medications.

  It appears with signs of systemic rheumatic disease:
  - ❖ *Fever, CNS* involvement (dizziness, spasms, clouded consciousness)
    - *Exanthem* (Chap. 9.1.1), *bleeding* (nasal, mucosal, gastrointestinal)
    - *Hepatosplenomegaly*
    - *Elevated CRP, ferritin, serum triglyceride level*; decreasing *ESR*
    - *Pancytopenia*
    - *Coagulopathy* (increased d-dimer levels and abnormal prothrombin time /PT/ and partial thromboplastin time /PTT/)

Bone marrow puncture, liver or *lymph node biopsy*: proof of *hemophagocytic macrophages* confirms the diagnosis.

(Auto) Immunological Phenomena and Serological Diagnostics

11

(Auto) immunological and immunomorphological phenomena, serological, and pathogen diagnostics, have no absolute specificity but in practice are of much importance.[12, 15, 21, 23] In this chapter, the most important information on rheumatology is presented in a practical way, as well as the possibilities and limitations are discussed.

11.1
Connective Tissue Disease (CTD) Serology

- *ANA* (*screening* test with indirect immunofluorescence in HEp-2 cells), *disease-unspecific*, often inappropriate also in older patients with no disease or in patients with fatigue or diffuse pain (think of fibromyalgia!)

ANA and *ENA* differentiation should then take place in order to identify more or less *disease-specific* and *sensitive* tests:

- *Systemic lupus erythematosus (SLE)*
  - *ANA, homogeneous* or *lightly speckled pattern of fluorescence*
    - ANA is positive in >95% of patients with *SLE* (usually be ELISA)
    - Negative ANA does not exclude the *SLE*
    - *ssDNA*-Ab, almost *always in SLE*, but *not disease-specific*
    - *dsDNA*-Ab, *disease-specific*/CS 27, 29, 34, 51, 71/(in ELISA, then confirmed by radioimmunoassay or Crithidia test), could predict or be associated with an episode, could be regressive under immunosuppression (CS 38)
  - *ENA* (will usually be checked for when ANA is positive)
    - *Nucleosomal* antibodies (in ELISA), *disease-specific*, both correlating to the activity of *SLE* (CS 27)
    - *Ribosomal* (against protein P) antibodies have high specificity and low sensitivity, associated with neuropsychiatric syndromes
    - *Sm*-Ab, *disease-specific* (*ACR* criterion), but not sensitive (in 10–30%), associated with *renal* and *CNS* involvement, correlated to *SLE activity* over the course
    - *U1-RNA*-Ab associated with prognostically favorable forms, *Raynaud's* syndrome and *myositis, not disease-specific* (only for *MCTD*)

E. Benenson, *Rheumatology*, Symptoms and Syndromes
DOI: 10.1007/978-1-84996-462-3_11, © Springer-Verlag London Limited 2011

- *SS-A(Ro)*-Ab associated with *sicca* syndrome, *neonatal lupus, photosensitization, arrhythmias* (specific for cardiac conducting tissue)
- *SS-B(La)*-Ab (the same clinical associations as with SSA-Ro)
- *Antiphospholipid* antibodies (Chap. 11.4)
- Low *complement C3* and *C4* level associated with disease activity
- *Coombs* test (particularly in *hemolytic anemia*)
- *Anti-thrombocytic* antibodies (in autoimmune thrombocytopenia, CS 28)
- *False-positive Wassermann* reaction (*cave* false *Syphilis* diagnosis).
- *Drug-induced lupus (DIL)*/Drugs implicated are *definitely:* procainamide, hydralazine, minocicline; *possible:* sulfasalazine, statins; *suggested:* multiple antibiotics, oral contraceptives, TNF – blockers/
  - *Histone*-Ab – selectively *positive* (in 75–95% of DIL, but in 75% of SLE)
  - *pANCA*
  - *dsDNA*-Ab *negative* but high frequency of *ssDNA*-Ab
  - *C3* and *C4* concentrations usually not decreased
- *Systemic sclerosis (SSc)*
  - ANA (a *nucleolar, homogeneous* or *patchy* pattern of fluorescence), if with a high titer, is suggestive of *SSc* and cannot always be differentiated (CS 16), prevalence >95%, *negative ANA* tends not to be typical of *SSc*, makes the diagnosis very unlikely
  - *ENA*
    - *Scl-70*-Ab (diffuse *SSc*, early organ involvement, rapid progression (CS 19, 54), could be the case with confirmed *SLE* (CS 51)
    - *Pm-Scl-70*-Ab characteristic of the diffuse form; the prognosis for patients with such a factor is better: higher rate of survival and less organ involvement
    - *Ribonucleoprotein* antibodies (*anti-U1RNP*), a risk factor for severe gastrointestinal involvement
    - *Centromere* antibodies/*anti-Cenp-Ab*/are typical of *limited SS* (CREST syndrome, CS 32, 58) associated with good survival, and not typical of *diffuse SSc*,
    - *Anti-RNA polymerase*-Ab a risk factor for scleroderma renal crisis
- *Polymyositis/dermatomyositis (PM/DM)*
  - *ANA (homogeneous or patchy pattern of fluorescence)*
  - *ENA* (about 30–40% of patients have following myositis-specific Ab)
    - *Mi2*-Ab (mostly in *DM*)
    - *Jo-1*-Ab (*anti-tRNA synthetase* Ab) associated with
      - *Antisynthetase* syndrome or clinical syndromes:
        - PM
        - Interstitial pulmonary involvement
        - *Arthritis*
        - *Raynaud's* syndrome
    - *SRP*-Ab (Ab to signal recognition particle) associated with necrotizing myopathy and treatment-refractory disease)
- *Mixed connective tissue disease (MCTD)*
  - *ANA, speckled pattern of fluorescence*
  - *ENA > 1:1600*/definitively *disease-specific*/

- *Ribonucleoprotein* antibodies (*anti*-U1RNP) without anti-Sm and without dsDNA-Ab (CS 2), absolute s*ensitivity* for *MCTD*
- *Sm*-Ab positive (an *exclusion criterion for this disease*)
- *PM-ScL*-Ab (associated with *PM/DM* and/or *SSc* symptoms)
- *Rheumatoid factors*
- *Sjögren's* syndrome (*primary*)/CS 18, 49, 53, 56/has a similar pattern
  - *ANA*/high-titer/
  - *ENA*
    - *SS-B/La*-Ab
    - *SS-A/Ro*-Ab (often combined with *La/SS-B*, occurring *also in SLE*)
  - *RF*, especially *IgA type* (DD *RA*, with mostly IgM type, and *cryoglobulinemia*)
  - *Hypergamma*- and *IgG-globulinemia*
- *Sjögren's* syndrome (*secondary*, e.g., in *RA, SSc* or *CREST* syndrome)
  - *ENA* (*SS-B/La* and *SS-A/Ro*) mostly not detectable
- *Lupus-associated hepatitis*
  - *ANA, ASMA*/anti-smooth muscle-Ab/and antimitochondrial-Ab (*AMA*)
- *Autoimmune hepatitis* or "*lupoid hepatitis*"
  - *ANA* and *ASMA* (Typ I)
  - *ALKM*-1/Ab to liver kidney microsomes/, *ALC*-1/Ab to liver cytosolic antigen/ (Typ II).
- *Autoimmune thyroiditis*/Hashimoto's (Chap. 12.4.4).
  - *ANA*, Ab to *thyroglobulin, thyroid-peroxidase* (TPO) and *thyroid microsomes.*

CTD serology was *absolutely pivotal* to the clinical interpretation (solutions discussed in → *RCS*, Chap. 2 and listed in the Appendix):

- *These findings confirm the diagnosis of CTD:*
  - In a female patient with *SLE* (Fig. 2) the diagnosis was changed to *MCTD* on account of ENA with *Anti-U1RNP*; clinical findings and lack of dsDNA-Ab are more likely associated with this disease.
  - Recurrent neurological and visual deficits, and *CNS* involvement (Fig. 50) were initially interpreted as *MS* despite high-titer ANA/up to 1: 32 000/for 3 years, and interferon treatment was administered. The more recently ascertained fluorescence pattern of ANA (*SS-B/La*- and *SS-A/Ro*-Ab) confirms the diagnosis. Do these findings, with such a set of symptoms (CS 18), enable diagnosis of an inflammatory rheumatic disease, and if so, which one?
  - Deformities of the hands consistent with *RA* (Fig. 70) are, in the presence of *anti-U1RNP*-Ab and absence of *anti-CCP*-Ab and *RF*, clearly to be interpreted as *MCTD* (CS 24).
  - In the case of serologically confirmed *SLE* (CS 29), there was an *acute* development of severe *abdominal pain*. Such rare complications (one incident of *ileus* and another of *renal venous thrombosis*) are easier to investigate serologically.
  - In a female patient with *sicca* syndrome and *MCP arthritis* (Fig. 89), *anti-centromere* and *anti-CCP*-Ab were found. So which diseases are present right now (CS 32)?

- *Acute hemolytic anemia* and *pneumonia* in a hospitalized female patient aged 25 years were judged to be associated with *Chlamydia*. *CTD* serology initiated somewhat later revealed an *SLE-specific* antibody profile (with the exception of *Scl-70-*Ab). Should the diagnosis be modified (CS 51)?
- A female patient with pain and swelling in the finger joints and high-titer *RF* was given treatment for some years/by me/for *seropositive RA*. Clinically, non-erosive *arthritis* and negative bone scintigraphy were remarkable. Could the high-titer *ENA* with *SS-A/Ro* and *SS-B/La* pattern be a better way of interpreting the full scope of the problems? (CS 53).
- *Query from a colleague*: "You have established a form of *CTD*, but how did you make that decision?" *CTD* serology (combined with *polyneuropathy, Raynaud's, sicca, myasthenic* syndrome and *esophageal motility disorders*) was pivotal. Her opinion on this finding: *ANA* 1:2 560, speckled pattern of fluorescence, *SS-A/Ro, RNP, Jo-1* detectable, *dsDNA*-Ab slightly positive, *Crithidia luciliae* negative (cf. CS 2).

- *The diagnosis of CTD was not confirmed* in the sense of the clinical findings despite detectable *ANA* or *dsDNA*:

  - Despite high-titer *ANA* and *ACLA*, with acute *thrombosis* of the *Aorta abdominalis* (Fig. 12) and *multi-infarct* syndrome in the *CNS* (Fig. 17), it was not *SLE* (lack of organ involvement and no dsDNA Ab), but rather *primary antiphospholipid* syndrome that was diagnosed.
  - In the case of acute *digital gangrene* (Fig. 47), the high-titer *ANA* in the absence of *dsDNA*-Ab and system/organ involvement is *more* indicative of *SSc* or *Buerger's* disease than of *SLE* (CS 16).
  - A 70-year-old male patient suffered several months of *fever, polyserositis,* elevated *CRP* and *dsDNA*-Ab (low titer), responding to cortisone and being discharged with the diagnosis of *SLE*. Is this diagnosis justified? Is there an alternative? (CS 62).
  - Persistent *B symptoms* with *fever, weight loss* should, in the case of low-titer ANA, be investigated and interpreted as *CTD* without any differentiation from other concepts (Fig. 74, CS 25).

- *CTD serology was* possibly not recorded or, in the context of clinical examinations, *inadequately assessed:*

  - In a 14-year-old male, *chorea* was understood to be associated with *rheumatic fever* (at the time, *SLE* immunology and *proteinuria* were not examined). After 3 years, periarticular swelling developed (Fig. 128c), *proteinuria* and true *lupus*-specific serology (see above) with *antiphospholipid* syndrome. Can the question – was it even *SLE* at the time? – be answered conclusively? (See *RCS*, Chap. 1.2.2).
  - A female patient suffered from the age of 16 from recurrent *mastitis, ANA-positive* (incidentally without dsDNA-Ab), *fatigue* and unexplained *feverish episodes*. Eight years later, due to organ involvement (exudative *pleuritis*, morphologically confirmed *LN*), *SLE* was established. Was the *ANA-positive mastitis* itself the first symptom of *SLE*? (CS 38).
  - In a female patient with acute *myelitis, mouth ulcers* and *Moschcowitz* syndrome (CS 64), low titers of ANCA were detected and the clinical picture initially interpreted as *vasculitis*. Is that correct?

11.1.1
RA Serology

- *CRP, ESR, fibrinogen* (acute-phase reaction) are *signs of activity*, but very *unspecific*; a lack of such parameters (prior to therapy) more or less complicates the diagnosis of "classic" *RA*, with the exception of oligoarthritic involvement
- *RF* (rheumatoid factors, IgM in ELISA) have approx. 80% specificity (see above), and approx. 70% sensitivity; up to 25% in the highest age group, but low titers
- *Anti-CCP*-Ab (against *c*yclic *c*itrullinated *p*eptide) are *sensitive* (up to 80%) for early diagnosis of *RA*, similar to *RF*, and *highly specific* (up to 97%) for *RA* versus *RF*-IgM. They could be detectable prior to clinical manifestation (up to 14 years) and are regarded as an *unfavorable prognostic factor*.

11.2
Vasculitis Serology

- *ANCA* (*screening* test with indirect immunofluorescence for neutrophils). A distinction is made between *ANCA-associated and* non-*ANCA associated vasculitis*
- *ANCA-associated vasculitis* (CS 12, 31, 48, 72, 73) (*Proteinase 3* as an important antigen for *cytoplasmic/cANCA/*staining, usually corresponds to presence of anti-proteinase-3 Ab/PR3-*ANCA*/, detected by ELISA; *myeloperoxidase* as an important antigen for *perinuclear/pANCA/*staining, usually corresponds to the presence of anti-myeloperoxidase Ab/MPO-*ANCA*/, detected by ELISA)
  - *Wegener's granulomatosis* (*WG*)/Figs. 75, 86, 96, 112/
    - *The presence of both a cANCA* has a *high positive predictive* value, is 70–90% sensitive for active generalized form *WG* compared with *inactive* initially (50% of cases), and *panarteritis nodosa* (10%); MPO-*ANCA* occurs in 10% of patients with *WG*
    - RF in the range 40–50%, associated with rheumatoid nodule-like granuloma ("Churg-Strauss granuloma"
  - *Churg–Strauss* syndrome (*CSS*)/CS 72/
    - *pANCA* in the range of 50%
    - *cANCA* (but not to both) 10%
    - RF associated with "Churg-Strauss granuloma"
  - *Microscopic polyangiitis* (*MPA*)/Fig. 33/
    - The combination of both a *pANCA* has a high positive value (in ca. 70%)
    - *cANCA* and PR3-*ANCA* in 40%
    - Anti-glomerular basement Ab
  - *Drug-induced ANCA-associated Vasculitis* frequently associated with very high titers of *pANCA*
  - *Rapid progressive glomerulonephritis* (*GN*), *pANCA* positive in 65%.
- *Non-ANCA-associated primary vasculitis* (CS 20)
  - *Classic panarteritis nodosa* (*PAN*)/Figs. 10–11/or *cutaneous forms* (Fig. 2), PAN is not considered to be an ANCA-associated vasculitis.
    - *pANCA* 15%

- *cANCA* 5–10%
- *Hepatitis B* antigen (in 40%) and *HCV* serology (in 20%) *positive*
- Absence of *ANA* and *dsDNA*-Ab
- *Henoch–Schönlein* purpura (*HSP*) – no serological markers, *IgA* immunocomplexes in the blood and in situ (on immunohistology)
- *Hypersensitivity vasculitis* (*HSV*) or *cutaneous leukocytoclastic angiitis* – no serological markers, may be diagnosed clinically and by biopsy
- *Urticarial Vasculitis* (the lesions persisted more than 24 h)
  - Normocomplementemic forms are likely to have a self-limited course, is viewed as a subset of *HSV*
  - Hypocomplementemic (serum C3, C4, and C1q levels are depressed) forms have many clinical similarities to *SLE*
  - Presence of anti-C1q-Ab (may be found in patients with *SLE*)
  - ANA without dsDNA-Ab, may have, if overlap with *SLE* is present
- *Behçet*'s disease produced no specific blood test abnormalities
- *Buerger*'s disease, there is no single diagnostic test
- *Cryoglobulinemic vasculitis* (*cry-V*)/Figs. 56ab/can be confirmed by the (serum) determination of *cryoglobulins*; they consist of antibodies (*Ig*), which become insoluble when cold and redissolve when heated (hence the serum specimens should be transported at a temperature of 37°C!) and possess the characteristics of *RF* or *cold agglutinins*, which are associated with varying etiologies (infections, autoimmune, or malignant diseases):
  - Type I: monoclonal IgG or IgM (it is more likely to be associated with syndromes of hyperviscosity and a hematopoietic malignancy, for example, NHL)
  - Type II: mixed, mostly monoclonal IgM and polyclonal IgG with *RF* activity, is often associated with low C4 complement levels and normal levels of C3
  - Type III: mixed polyclonal immunoglobulins, mostly IgM

Vasculitis associated with Typ II and III involves both small (more common)-and medium-sized blood vessels, it is caused by hepatitis C virus, the development of *cry-V* occurs in only a small minority.

When analyzing *vasculitis serology*, the clinical findings are a priority:

- Positive findings can confirm the clinical diagnosis, especially *WG* (versus, e.g., *PAN*), whereby *cANCA* is highly specific and sensitive
- *pANCA* is more specific and sensitive for *CSS, MPA, drug-induced vasculitis* (very high titers), and *rapid progressive glomerulonephritis*
- With other forms of *vasculitis* and low ANCA titers, such immunological findings should not be overestimated, as was the case in CS 64
- Negative serology does not on the whole rule out vasculitis (CS 11)
- It must be noted thereby that more than *half of all cases of vasculitis* are attributable to the subgroup of *undifferentiated vasculitis* (as shown, in my opinion, in Figs. 30–32)
- Hypocomplementemic finding associated with *urticarial vasculitis*
- *Cry-V* has almost specific immunological pattern (s. above)

- Several forms of *vasculitis* do not absolutely have any immunological markers:
  - Each of the *large* vessels
  - Some of the *medium-vessel* as *Buerger's*, and *primary CNS vasculitis*
  - *Small-vessel vasculitis* as *HSP, Behçet's, hypersensitivity vasculitis*
- Consequently, the immunological data from *vasculitis*, which are not always detectable, play a subordinate role to morphology and radiology
- In the *follow-up*, such findings play only a limited role: potentially *cANCA* in *WG*, cryoglobulins in *cry-V*

11.3
Pathogen and Serological Diagnostics

Such diagnostic methods should always be instigated if diseases exist, which, clinically, are suspected to be associated with infections. Primarily, *pharyngeal, enteral, and urogenital infections* are concerned, which could induce *rheumatic fever* (rarely in Germany), most commonly *ReA* and in a minority of cases *SpA*. The problems with *Borrelia* antibodies and the known or suspected *viral* conditions with *hepatitis B, C*, and *HIV*, are everyday issues – some examples are given from our patient population.

11.3.1
Rheumatic Fever

Rheumatic fever is a systemic, immune-mediated disease, which is triggered by infection with group A *streptococci*. The disease is rather unlikely to occur without a prior streptococcal infection (pharyngeal, angina, scarlet fever) and *imminent* increase in *Streptococci* antibodies (anti-streptolysin O and other anti-streptococcal antibody). If acquired valvular defects (particularly mitral stenosis can be replaced by valvular regurgitation) there is often no history.

The diagnostic difficulties with a 16-year-old female patient with rheumatic fever are seen in the following case (CS 71): this disease was diagnosed three years ago, initially due to *Chorea minor* (incidentally, 9 months – far too long! – after *pharyngeal infection*). At the same time, *polyarthralgia* with no *carditis* and *serologically* elevated anti-streptolysin O-Ab were found.

Three years later, *polyarthralgia* also developed with pain-free swelling of individual joints (Fig. 128c), massive *proteinuria, antiphospholipid* syndrome, and *dsDNA*-Ab, also confirmed by *Crithidia test*, and again slightly elevated anti-streptolysin O-Ab.

So it is justifiable to question whether this case involved two inflammatory rheumatic diseases or only *SLE*. Whatever the case, the *Jones criteria* of rheumatic fever were in fact fulfilled/one major criterion and two minor criteria/but they were not related in time to the *pharyngeal infection* (*Chorea* 9 months after infection!) and the anti-streptolysin O-Ab were elevated, in fact, at the point when *SLE* developed and was confirmed by all criteria.

11.3.2
Yersinia-Induced Arthritis

Yersinia-induced arthritis (CS 36, 37, 60, 69) is also to be approached as a diagnostic challenge:

- *Clinically*, by a *pattern of involvement untypical of RA* (asymmetric *oligoarthritis* of the large and small joints, unstable, RF and anti-CCP-Ab negative) affecting the soft-tissue structures, namely, *tendinitis, enthesitis* (Fig. 102) or even with *isolated* heel pain and *plantar fasciitis* (Fig. 98), or to begin with months of *fever*, increased *CRP*, and also *polyarthritis* (CS 60) or *sacroiliitis* (in *HLA-B27* positive patients with a history of disc problems, CS 69) or *Erythema nodosum* (Fig. 109).
- *Serologically*, the detection of *fresh Yersinia infection* in these patients was indicative on *immunoblot* and *ELISA*, namely, the detection of *IgA* Ab, which incidentally could persist for years (CS 37). The suffered infection is indicated by the detection of *IgG*.

The serological aspects should, when making a diagnosis, be *secondary to the clinical factors*, such as in this case (CS 60): To begin with, there was a *septicemic-typhous pattern* to *Yersinia* infection with *IgA* antibodies lasting for several months. Later, a pathological picture emerged, which now can be interpreted rather as *seronegative RA* than as *ReA* on account of the stable arthritis in the large (with wrist) and some small (MCP, PIP) joints. This is indicated, in my opinion, also on account of the inefficacy of 3 years of therapy (MTX, Arava®, Decortin®, Remicade® three times, rituximab, several RSO).

- *Detection of pathogens* in the feces (only 1–2 weeks after onset of symptoms) could also lead to administration of antibiotics, which in *arthritis* and the proof of *IgA* Ab is not advisable.
- The *course* was recurrent and chronic in almost 50% (of all the patients mentioned above), but there was no development of *SpA*.

11.3.3
Chlamydia-Induced Arthritis

Chlamydia-induced arthritis is not a serological, but rather a clinical diagnosis. Attention must be paid, in particular, to:

- *Chlamydia infection* (C. trachomatis) belongs to *sexually transmitted diseases* with the risk of other, more serious infections (gonococcal, among others) and with C. Trachomatis-associated common syndromes (males: urethritis, epididymitis; females: cystitis/urethritis, acute pelvic inflammatory, ulcerative lesions of the genitalia)
- *Historical evidence* (genitourinary infections usually occurring due to a new sexual partner, often progressing asymptomatically in women, and lasting up to a few weeks)

- *Typical pattern of joint involvement*, namely, *oligoarthritis*, mostly *arthritis* of the knee (as in Fig. 25) or hotspots in the finger joints or *dactylitis* (one patient was also found to have *episcleritis*, recurrent *enthesiopathy* and serologically confirmed C.trachomatis infection). One HLA-B27-positive patient with *Chlamydia-induced arthritis* developed typical *SpA* (as in Figs. 117, 124)
- *Serological proof* is suitable more for screening due to a lack of specificity and sensitivity, whereby IgM Ab can be detected more in the early phase, and then IgG (in 2–4 weeks). Only a titer elevation is of diagnostic relevance
- *Direct proof of pathogens* (smears for genitourinary infection, morning urine by means of *ELISA or PCR*). In such a case the sexual partner should also be treated
- *Chlamydia pneumoniae* has only recently been recognized as an arthritis-inducing pathogen, but can trigger *pneumonia*, as initially suspected in one of our cases (CS 51). Combined with *hemolytic anemia* on the basis of the serological data, the finding was evidently interpreted too directly, with a typical pattern of *SLE* emerging thereafter.

11.3.4
Borrelia Arthritis or Lyme Borreliosis

This tick-transmitted spirochetal illness often poses a tremendous diagnostic problem in everyday rheumatology, particularly on detection of *Borrelia burgdorferi* Ab and nonspecific symptoms, such as *fatigue* or *arthralgia* (DD *fibromyalgia)*, which should not always be followed up. Unnecessary antibiotic therapy could thus be avoided. On the other hand, due to the clinical heterogeneity of the disease – as suspected in our case – many cases may be overlooked or diagnosis may involve a certain degree of uncertainty, mostly on the part of the patients. The diagnosis of *borreliosis* is mainly a *clinical problem* due to the following factors:

- *Epidemiological data* (epidemic region and tick bite elicitable only in approximately 30% of those exposed) should be examined closely
- *Course* or *stages* of the disease should be established after an incubation period of 3–32 days above all:
  - *Erythema chronicum migrans* (circular, macular skin changes with the tick bite in the center) regressing after approximately 4 weeks; concurrent "flu-like"or "meningitis-like" symptoms (stage I)
  - *Lymphocytoma* of the skin (*Lymphadenitis cutis benigna*, Fig. 20a), the typical pattern is migratory pain in joints, tendons, bursae, muscle, or bone, usually without joint swelling or *arthritis, dactylitis,* or *enthesiopathy*, possibly *CNS (facial paresis, meningitis, myelitis)*, ocular (*uveitis*), and *cardiac* (AV-block, *peri/-myocarditis)* involvement (stage II)
  - *Oligoarthritis* (chronic *gonarthritis*, among others), *Acrodermatitis chronica atrophicans, CNS, ocular,* and *cardiac* symptoms (stage III)
  - *Serology* is *mostly positive in those affected*, but could also be *positive in those who are not sick*

- *Screening* test with ELISA and immunofluorescence for determining antibodies to *B. burgdorferi* in the serum: specific IgM-Ab is already detectable at stage I, IgG-Ab tend almost always to be detectable in stages II–III
- Specification of such findings by immunoblot (western blot): antibodies against antigens 23 kD, 39 kD, 41 kD, and certain other types are specific for IgM and IgG[15]
- Pathogen detection with PCR is not yet suitable for routine diagnostics

11.4
Antiphospholipid Syndrome

Antiphospholipid syndrome(*APS*) is an acquired hypercoagulable state, the most common cause of *thrombophilia* and presents in the form of

- *Peripheral arterial occlusion*, recurrent venous, and more rarely, arterial *thrombosis*, even in aortic *Leriche* syndrome (Fig. 12), and *embolism*, and should be confirmed by angiogram, MRI, Doppler sonography or histology (occlusion of individual subcutaneous vessels):
  - *Skin*: *Livedo reticularis* or *racemosa* (Figs. 2, 20a, 30–31), necrotic purpura, gangrene (as in Fig. 47)
  - *Lower extremities* (most often deep vein thrombosis) or large veins (*Axillaris, Subclavia, Cava inferior*): *phlebothrombosis*
  - *Pulmonary embolism* in roughly a third of patients with *phlebothrombosis*
  - *Pulmonary thrombosis, primary*
  - *CNS*: in this case more *arterial thrombosis* with seizures, transitory ischemic attacks, cerebral insults (Fig. 17), cerebral venous sinus thrombosis; epilepsy, migraine, *Amaurosis fugax*
  - *Heart*: *ischemic and valvular* heart diseases, early bypass occlusions
  - *Kidneys*: thrombotic microangiopathy, venous thrombosis (CS 29), arterial stenosis
- High *rate of recurrent thrombosis* (up to 30%)
- *Habitual miscarriages* (early, before the *10th week of pregnancy*) due to placental vascular occlusion
- *Thrombocytopenia* and potentially *hemolytic anemia* (CS 64)
- *Antiphospholipid* or *anticardiolipin* antibodies (*ACLA*): isotype IgG associated with *arterial thrombosis, ACLA*-IgM with *spontaneous miscarriages* and thrombocytopenia, *lupus anticoagulant* with *venous thrombosis*). *ACLA* alone is not sufficient for *APS* diagnosis (CS 38)
- *Lupus anticoagulant, PTT*/partial thromboplastin time/prolongation (clearly confirm diagnosis of *APS*, CS 71), but occur frequently in infections, some types of tumors
- *ACLA* against ß2-glycoprotein I (IgG, IgM)

To confirm *APS*, a repeat test is required for *ACLA* at an interval of at least *12 weeks* along with at least *one clinical criterion*. At the same time, *CTD* serology should be instigated in order to be able to distinguish between the *forms of APS*:

- *Primary* (disease or *Sneddon's* syndrome)/CS 3, 6/
- *Secondary* (developed, e.g., from *CTD,* about 50% have *SLE*/CS 71/or *vasculitis*)

'*Catastrophic*' or '*fatal*' *APS* in *disseminated* thrombosis with *multiorgan failure* (*renal failure, CNS* involvement/Fig. 17/), or peripheral *gangrene* (as in Fig. 47) or *acute Leriche* syndrome (Fig. 12, CS 3); the acute occlusion of the aorta may occur as the result of in situ thrombosis in a preexisting severely narrowed segment of the aorta[7] as part of a vasculitis without the APS, both lower extremities were amputated at the lines of demarcation due to the development of higher peripheral gangrene (Fig. 132).

11.5
T- and B- Activation and Dysregulation

At the present time, these *immunological* processes represent the *pathophysiological basis* and primary concern of practice-oriented rheumatology research (ACR, EULAR congresses). They form a largely identified network of *activated T, B, NK cells* and osteoclasts, which produce the *pro-inflammatory* (TNF-alpha, IL-1, IL-6, IL-17, IL-23 and many others) and *anti-inflammatory* (soluble TNF-receptor molecules, IL-1RA, IL-2r, IL-10) cytokines as well as *RF* and thus, on the one hand, actuate immunological inflammation and bone destruction while on the other hand possibly limiting such processes.

Such processes have been researched in *RA* but also in *AS* and *PsA* with such success during the last decade that different targets in the cytokine network and related antagonists have been detected and genetically engineered. Such medications (*biologicals*) significantly expand or even *revolutionize* the therapeutic possibilities in *severe, treatment-resistant cases* of these and other inflammatory diseases – namely, with *curative* approaches (e.g., in early-onset *RA*) – or they may achieve *remission* or a drug-free state. Such promising options have a highly favorable useful/side effect profile, but do have enormous economic and socioeconomic consequences.

The *new objectives* in rheumatology have been made possible by the following *biologicals*, some of which are approved or are undergoing preclinical and clinical testing (see too Chap. 7.3.2):

- *Monoclonal antibodies* against TNF-alpha (Remicade®/*infliximab*, Humira®/*adalimubab*), approved as a *first line* therapy for *RA, AS, PsA, plaque psoriasis, Crohn's* disease, *Colitis ulcerosa*, mostly in combination with MTX)
- The second generation of these agents is

- Cimzia®/*certolizumab pegol* (approved as a first line therapy for *RA*)
- Simponi®/*golimumab* a human anti-TNF monoclonal antibody (approved as a *first line* therapy for *RA, AS, PsA*)
- *Soluble TNF-alpha receptor inhibitors*, aimed at blocking the potentially damaging effect of such receptors (Enbrel®/*etanercept*), approved for the aforementioned articular, spinal and skin diseases, and *JIA*, also as *monotherapy*
- *Interleukin-1 blockers*
  - *Receptor antagonist* (IL-1RA, Kineret®/*anakinra*)
  - *Antibodies* against these cytokines (Ilaris®/*canakinumab*), which approved for treatment of some autoinflammatory diseases and syndrome (e.g., *CAPS*: Muckle-Wells, Familial Cold Autoinflammatory; Still's and *gout*→Chap. 8.1)
  - *Dimeric fusion protein, rilonacept*
- *IL-6 receptor blocker* (RoActemra®/*tocilizumab*, a recently approved substance for *first line* and monotherapy for *RA*)
- *Antibodies against CD20*/B-cells/(Mabthera®/*rituximab*), approved for *second line* therapy in TNF-resistant *RA* patients
- *Antibodies* against *CD19* (*ocrelizumab*) are currently in phase 3 development
- First *selective T-cell co-stimulation modulator* (Orencia®/*abatacept*), approved as *first line* therapy for RA patient and for JIA.
- CP-690, 550 Tasocitinib® is being developed as a first nonbiological DMARD for the treatment of *RA* and other, inflammatory conditions, is a selective inhibitor of the Janus kinase (JAK); the resultant suppression of T-, B-, and NK-cell function is highly effective (currently in phase 3 development).

All these medications have been clinically tested (Department of Internal Medicine, investigator Dr A Rubbert) within the framework of marketing authorization studies, and are currently in use.

Immunological activities for the purposes of diagnosis and follow-up most often cover, in practice, the following cell parameters:

- Number of T- and B-cells (question of existing immune defect or control of *B-cell depletion* in RA therapy with *rituximab*)
- T-cell activation by
  - HLA-DR4 (associated with poor prognosis for RA)
  - T-cell cytokines or interleukins (IL) – serum measurements (TNF-alpha, IL-1, IL-2r, IL-6)
- B-activation
  - *Increased* Ig concentration (for diagnosis of an immune defect, e.g., some forms of *CTD, Sjögren's* syndrome and therapeutic monitoring)
  - *Increased circulating immune complexes*
  - *(Auto) antibody hyperproduction*, above all *RF, ANA* (Chap. 11).

11.6
Immunomorphological Syndromes

When using *bone marrow puncture, skin, muscle, organ biopsies* (Chap. 13.9), these are a means of *invasive diagnostics* and represent the next *diagnostic opportunity*. Below, the scope – though not to the full extent – and specific clinical significance of morphological diagnostics are outlined:

- *Bone marrow biopsy* for
  - *Unclear diagnosis* with *B symptoms, lymphadenopathy and hepatolienal* syndrome, for example, in *Still's* disease (CS 62), *Sjögren's* syndrome (CS 56)
  - *Cytopenia* in *SLE, RA* under intensified immunosuppression (CS 68) while querying whether it is related to disease or medication
  - *Secondary cryoglobulinemic vasculitis, monoclonal gammapathy*, and suspected *plasmocytoma* (was therefore excluded in Fig. 132).
- *Skin/muscle biopsies* on suspicion of
  - *PM/DM* (a primary criterion), *SLE* (Fig. 20, no finding; in a female patient with clinically and immunologically confirmed *Sjögren's* syndrome, CS 49, *lupus* was diagnosed morphologically; the morphological diagnosis is not disease-specific), *sarcoidosis* (Figs. 83, 90 confirmed the diagnosis)
  - *SSc* (*distal gangrene*, Fig. 47) with high-titer ANA and no differentiation, whereby the morphological finding was not indicative
  - *SLE*, clinically confirmed (CS 64, see comments in *RCS*, Chap. 2), DD *vasculitis*. *Skin biopsy*: fibrosis, sclerosis, discrete lymphocytic infiltrates (more likely consistent with *SSc*, not a typical pattern for *SLE*)
  - *Vasculitis* in:
    - Existing *polyneuropathy* (CS 72), confirming, morphologically, the diagnosis of "*Churg-Strauss granulom*" (rheumatoid-like cutaneous extravascular necrotizing granuloma) (Chap. 11.2)
    - Subcutaneous *nodes* of unknown origin (Fig. 33) whereby *microscopic polyangiitis/MPA/*was diagnosed
    - *Ulcer* with *Livedo racemosa*, whereby in one case (Fig. 2) *Panarteritis nodosa/PAN/*was confirmed; in the other, clinically similar but more pronounced case (Figs. 30–31), none of the 3 biopsies revealed a morphological correlate of *PAN*; hence this last case should, in my opinion, be described as *undifferentiated vasculitis* or *vasculopathy*
    - *Henoch–Schönlein* purpura/*HSP*/revealed very specifically the *IgA*-containing deposits of immune complexes and complement
    - *Hypersensitivity vasculitis* (Fig. 113) confirmed the diagnosis
    - *Drug-induced* efflorescences (Figs. 110–111ab, 129b), in this case *Psoriasis pustulosa*

- \ Skin changes of unclear origin with Borrelia antibodies and response to tetra-cyclines (Fig. 20a) – not indicative
- Female patient suffering from *Leriche* syndrome 16 years ago (Fig. 12) presently developed *Livedo-type* skin changes morphologically consistent with *antiphospholipid* syndrome.
- *Organ biopsies* with involvement of
  - *Kidneys* with marked *nephrotic* syndrome of unclear etiology, or for estimating the activity and sclerotic index and prognosis (*classification* for *lupus nephritis*) under immunosuppressive therapy (Figs. 92–93)
  - *Lungs* in unclear disseminated *pulmonary fibrosis* and extensive shadowing on suspicion of *CTD* or *vasculitis* (Fig. 79- *histiocytosis X*)
  - *Lungs* (DD on suspicion of *tumors* or *rheumatoid nodules* (CS 13), *Pneumocystis carinii pneumonia*, particularly in immunosuppressed patients, *alveolitis*
  - *Liver* (in *hepatomegaly*/CS 69/, high liver values, with suspected *granulomatous hepatitis*, DD *autoimmune hepatitis*, and *SLE*)
  - *Heart* (DD between inflammatory and atherosclerotic changes in *cardiomyopathy*).
    - *Lymph nodes.* As a rule, no biopsy should be done in the case of *SLE*, *Still's* (CS 66) or *Sjögren's* syndrome (CS 49); since *lymphadenopathy* is part of the clinical picture, but often it has been done – as in our cases – in order to rule out *lymphoma*
    - *Salivary gland* (on suspicion of *lymphoma* as part of *Sjögren's* syndrome/CS 56/, with diagnosis thereby of *MALT lymphoma*)
    - *Joints* (biopsy is a routine procedure with arthroscopy and surgery)

Bones (Figs. 36b and 37) – initially deemed to be *TB* on account of the existing *granulomatous inflammation*; at present these changes (see in *RCS* CS 13, Chaps. 1.1.2 and 2) are regarded as *rheumatoid nodules*.

Treatment-Induced and Associated Conditions and Diseases

12

The use of all older and newer medications, from glucocorticoids to *biologicals*, is considerably limited by the adverse effects as well as by conditions and illnesses that already exist or emerge during therapy. Months or years of therapy with no adverse effects and without the new development of conditions and illnesses (as in Figs. 110–111, 129b) does not exactly sound very realistic, but should always be the aim. However, the downside to our therapeutic regimens, which can be described as "iatrogenic comorbidity," is relatively well known and should, therefore, be individually predicted and monitored, as well as actively prevented.

12.1
Glucocorticoid Therapy

Glucocorticoid is essential but may cause adverse effects, which are unavoidable and almost inevitable:

- *Osteoporosis* (Chap. 3.11.1, CS 46)
  - Back pain (Chap. 2.1)
  - Fracture, stress fractures, and/or sintering
  - Vertebral sintering due to collapsed vertebrae with *compression* syndrome (Figs. 125–127)
  - Dynamics of diminished bone density (by DEXA) and prophylactic therapy (Ca + vit. D)
- *Osteonecrosis, aseptic* (Chap. 3.10.1; Fig. 121, CS 44)
- *Diabetes mellitus* (CS 33)
  - Cortisone therapy should be reduced relatively rapidly at the first signs (HbA1c > 6.5%) and preferably stopped altogether
  - *Safe cortisone doses* (Decortin® to a maximum of 7.5 mg day) should be the aim
  - The disease must be treated at the same time (after consulting an endocrinologist)
- *Cushing* syndrome
  - Facial changes and *fatty deposits* ("buffalo neck"), *Striae rubrae*
  - *Weight gain* should be compensated for by dietary measures
  - *Arterial hypertension* should be treated routinely

E. Benenson, *Rheumatology*, Symptoms and Syndromes
DOI: 10.1007/978-1-84996-462-3_12, © Springer-Verlag London Limited 2011

- *Increased risk of infection* (CS 27) is more likely, hence glucocorticoids should always be combined with basic preparations and *biologicals* for the purposes of rapid reduction
- *Adrenal insufficiency* (if reduction is not optimal or abrupt discontinuation)

12.2
Conventional Immunosuppressive Therapy

Conventional immunosuppressive therapy (See Chap. 7.3.1, CS 70), or basic therapy takes priority in the treatment of inflammatory rheumatic diseases and is covered on all bases in specialist literature.[12, 14, 15] I have just a few practical comments from my experience. Prior to adjustment, thorough consideration should first be given to indications and contraindications, especially existing diseases (no serious concomitant diseases) and conditions (alcohol abuse), the desire to have children (comes first!) and compliance issues (trust and reliability of the patients are two of the most important requirements).

Basic therapy must also be adjusted very specifically to organ involvement and immunological activity in the case of *CTD* and *vasculitis*.

On one hand, persistent intensive immunosuppressive therapy, known as basic therapy, is to be viewed as unavoidable. When discontinuing or even reducing the treatment, a flare in one of these diseases can be expected at any time. On the other hand, during such therapy, adverse effects, which are often unavoidable, and even fatal complications can be expected:

- *Acquired (secondary) immune defect* (CS 38) with a tendency toward *persistent recurrent infections* of any nature, as far as *sepsis* (such a condition arose with acute renal failure immediately following tooth extraction in a 27-year-old woman with *RA*, but no concomitant diseases, who had been given a biologic/rituximab/3 months previously)
- *Bone marrow insufficiency* presenting as *cytopenia* (CS 68, DD *Felty's* syndrome)

12.3
Anti-cytokine Therapy

Anti-cytokine therapy for *RA, AS, PsA, plaque psoriasis, JIA, Crohn's disease, Colitis ulcerosa* (see Chap. 7.3.2) mostly administered at a weight-related dosage (except Enbrel®) using the following *biologicals* (the specific indication should be checked with each medication):

- Soluble TNF-alpha receptor fusion protein Enbrel®/*etanercept*, 25/50 mg *SC* twice or once per week
- TNF-alpha antibodies, monoclonal
  - Remicade®/*infliximab* infusion 2–5 mg/kg for about 1–2 h on weeks 0, 2, then at 6–8 weeks intervals
  - Humira®/*adalimubab*, 40 mg *SC* once every 2 weeks
  - Simponi®/*golimumab*, fully human antibody, 50 mg *SC* every 4 weeks
  - Cimzia®/*certolozumab*, 400 mg or 200 mg *SC* once every 2 weeks

- IL-6 receptor blocker (RoActemra®/*tocilizumab*), 8 mg/kg every 4 weeks, infusion 45 min
- IL-1Ra antagonists (Kineret®/*anakinra*), 100 mg *SC* daily
  - IL-1Ra-mAb (Ilaris®/*canakinumab*), 2 mg/kg or 150 mg *SC* every 8 weeks
- CD20/B-cells/Ab (Mabthera®/*rituximab*, *1,000–1,200 mg*, 2 infusions over 4–5 h within 2 weeks, then at 6–18-month intervals)
- First selective T-cell co-stimulation modulator (Orencia®/*abatacept*), 10 mg/kg, infusion 30 min at in 2 and 4 weeks, then every 4 weeks

Such an innovative and rather costly therapy should be initiated and administered under certain preconditions.[12, 14, 15, 23] For therapeutic recommendations, see Chap. 7.3.

We have learned from general, and our own, experience that such medications are highly effective if combined with other basic medications (registered with MTX) – except for Enbrel®, which is approved for monotherapy – thereby potentiating their immunosuppressive effect and avoiding adverse, but already known, side effects (possibly as a result of antibody formation, which has been proven during the use of Remicade® and Humira®). According to experience, such medications are tolerated very well and cause hardly any allergic reactions (with the exception of anakinra, with *panniculitis* at the injection site/ Fig. 16/; cortisone injection is proposed prior to rituximab infusion).

What is clinically relevant with such therapy is the exclusion of chronic infections, especially *hepatitis B, C, HIV,* and *TB*. Appropriate serological tests are necessary, as well as *Tine (SC)* and possibly *QuantiFERON* (in vitro) tests, and chest X-ray when adjusting TNF-blockers. Sometimes, as in one of our cases (CS 13), an in vitro *QuantiFERON* test should be carried out in addition to the *Tine* test (proved negative twice) in the event of morphological diagnosis of *bone TB*, Fig. 36b (at present, this diagnosis has been revised by experts in the direction of *RA*-specific changes). Furthermore, Enbrel® proves beneficial in this family with respect to increase in *TB* and other infections.

New *infections* (respiratory tract, urinary tract, CNS, e.g., progressive multifocal *leukoencephalopathy/PML/*) can be regarded as possible side effects of such therapies, but occur relatively rarely and should be treated with intensive antibiotic regimens. Once the complications have healed, the *biologics* should be continued, as necessary. If such infections recur, therapy should be discontinued or switched (e.g., to anakinra). Other rare complications from TNF-blockers are the new onset of *pustular psoriasis* (2 cases in our population, Figs. 110–111, 129b; a total of 120 cases of *pustular psoriasis* have been found with TNF blockers[27]) or *septic arthritis* in TEP of the knee joint, or *sepsis* with acute renal failure 3 months after rituximab infusion, in a 27-year-old woman with *RA* and no concomitant illness.

12.4
Associated Conditions and Diseases

Such situations more often pose clinically relevant problems than the underlying diseases themselves, possibly having a serious impact on *general health* and basic therapy. It is therefore important to recognize such problems as early as possible, as well as prevent and treat them adequately. They include *acute* (pneumonia, urinary tract infections, sepsis) and *chronic* (*TB* – an exclusion criterion, e.g., in TNF-blocker therapy) *infections, post-tumorous conditions*, adverse effects from previous and ongoing therapy, arising *complications* (e.g., intestinal infarctions in ANCA-positive *vasculitis*/CS 48/or *ileus* and acute *renal thrombosis* in *SLE*/CS 29/or conditions post *myocardial* or *cerebral infarctions*, CS 6) or unfortunately *iatrogenically induced states* (e.g.,/CS 38/*acute renal failure* in a patient with *SLE* having received high-dose ciclosporin therapy and in whom an ovarian cyst ruptured at the same time as a result of marcumar therapy, with suspected *APS*, which, over the course, could not be confirmed). Or paraplegia as a result of *cortisone-induced osteoporosis* with vertebral fracture (CS 46).

Where *lymphomas* and other tumors are concerned, there has, to date, been no significant incidence under the use of TNF-alpha blockers and other *biologics*. Since 2006, there have been nine cases in all of hepatosplenic *T-cell NHLs* registered under Remicade® (combined with azathioprine in *Crohn's* disease) and Humira® (in *RA*).

12.4.1
Chronic Hepatitis B and C

Viral diagnostics are obsolete if systemic *vasculitis* is suspected. *Chronic hepatitis B* (antigenemia/*HBsAg*/with immune complex development) and *chronic hepatitis C* are closely associated with *panarteritis nodosa* (*Hbs* positivity in 10–50%/<10% in the developed world/, a diagnostic criterion, *HVC* positivity in 20%). *Hepatitis C virus* infections (detection of Ab to HCV or HCV RNA) are closely associated with approximately 90% of all cases of *mixed cryoglobulinemia*/types II and III/ (Fig. 56, CS 20).

12.4.2
Atherosclerosis

This has recently come to be viewed as a variant of *chronic vasculitis*, with the elevation in *CRP* typical of the inflammatory rheumatic disease seen as a *trigger* for the inflammation. With a progressive course, *atherosclerosis* accelerates the increased mortality of our patients suffering primarily from *RA* and *CTD* by means of *cardiovascular diseases* and complications. Thus, the late sequelae of the diseases and most common causes of death, after more than 5–10 years of the disease, appear, e.g., in *SLE*.[20] In a recent meta-analysis, the risk of cardiovascular death was 50% higher in patients with *RA* when compared with the general population.

In some cases, the two causes (*coronaritis* and *atherosclerosis*) are suspected, e.g., in *myocardial infarction*, as in CS 26 of a 73-year-old male patient with *Behçet's* disease but no further risk factors for *coronary artery disease*. A typical pattern for *myocardial infarction* is to be questioned thereby on account of extremely elevated *CRP* and *ESR* (after the event) and complete regression of the symptoms from cortisone therapy.

In all events, the potential atherosclerotic factors in our patients with *CTD* and *vasculitis* should be closely monitored (clinical, lab measurements, ECG, Doppler sonography), namely:

- Metabolic disorders
- Arterial hypertension, obesity
- Problems with diabetes, particularly during
- Long-term maintenance therapy with glucocorticoids, which could merely potentiate such problems (but also possible adverse effects involving the eyes, gastrointestinal tract)

Such concomitant diseases and conditions should be treated appropriately and adequately, e.g., statin prescription even in young women with *SLE* (CS 38) or with *Takayasu's arteritis* (CS 21) which, however, could trigger a condition similar to *polymyalgia rheumatica* (Chap. 9.6.4).

12.4.3
HIV Infection

Such an infection presents a broad spectrum of rheumatological factors. Initially, the *general syndromes* are virtually the same (Chap. 8), and there is an increased incidence of rheumatological syndromes:

- Connective tissue:
  - Stubborn, stable, and possibly virus-induced *arthralgia*, but with *no radiological correlate* (X-ray, bone scintigram), and minimal response to NSAIDs
  - Increased occurrence of *arthritis* (Fig. 68) or *Tietze's* syndrome (Fig. 69) or *drumstick fingers* with *hour-glass nails* (Fig. 88) or stable *polyarthralgia* in the event of a positive family history of *psoriasis* – all such cases best fit into the concept of *psoriatic arthropathy* (CS 23) *sine psoriasis*. *De novo psoriasis* has a poor prognosis (CS 23). Moreover, *psoriasis* may appear initially or an existing case deteriorates considerably
  - Rare syndromes, e.g., *periostitis*, confirmed by MRI (with severe pain in one shin, own observation); *septic arthritis* and *osteomyelitis* have also been described
  - *PM-type* clinical pattern, possibly *pyomyositis* (could also be induced by medication and/or opportunistic infections/toxoplasmosis)
- *Organ* and *vascular involvement*
  - *Nephropathy*, a rapid progressive form, possibly with *SLE*-type morphology
  - *Sjögren's* syndrome (Chap. 10.7)
  - *Vasculitis* of the small (*hypersensitivity vasculitis*, *CNS* vasculitis) or medium-sized (*panarteritis nodosa*) vessels

12.4.4
Autoimmune Thyroiditis, Hypothyroidism

Autoimmune thyroiditis often associated with *CTD* and *vasculitis*, e.g., with *SSc* (in 25%).

A 30-year-old female patient with *Scl-70*-positive *SSc* (CS 54) developed a pronounced *polymyositis* syndrome with *myalgia, myasthenia*, and extreme *fatigue*, and *elevated CK* (up to factor 20). At the same time, she had extremely high *TSH* levels (up to factor 100). Only over the course was it possible – while simultaneously estimating such symptoms based on the thyroid values – to distinguish these conditions, namely, *polymyositis* syndrome as part of *SSc* or *hypothyroidism*. Adequate therapy with *L-thyroxine* (150 μg/day) returned the *TSH* values to within the normal range, but the *myalgia* and *increased CK* remained clinically relevant. Hence, the *myositis* syndrome as part of *SSc* seems certain.

Autoimmune thyroiditis could also develop in association with *CREST* syndrome (CS 58) and *vasculitis*, as in one of our cases with *hepatitis C*-induced *cryoglobulinemic vasculitis* (CS 20). Such patients must be treated with sometimes high, sometimes low *L-thyroxine* doses while monitoring the *TSH* concentrations.

Autoimmune thyroiditis should not be forgotten when evaluating high *ANA* values with no specific pattern of fluorescence, which has often been attributed to *SLE* or *SSc*. In such a case, the ANA, mostly with no particular pattern, is most likely of no clinical significance. The concurrent *arthralgia, myalgia* and *fatigue* with stable, normal TSH are more consistent with *fibromyalgia*.

For the purposes of nosological classification of *CTD* and *vasculitis*, it is imperative to use a comprehensive, general therapeutic approach, which extends far beyond the boundaries of one specialization, including all internal and other clinical specialties.[12, 14, 15, 21] In principle, any clinical symptom of these non-rheumatic diseases, *without exception*, could equally be a symptom of *CTD* and/or *vasculitis*. This variety and vague specificity of symptoms consequently makes the diagnostic pathway *from symptom to diagnosis* more difficult. One route, presented in this book, is to construct *diagnostic blocks*, i.e., *syndromes* and correlate them to one another. At the same time, the *causal, morphological, and immunological factors* need to be considered.[2]

While the diagnosis of *CTD* and *vasculitis* is known to be one of the most difficult in internal medicine, it is an attainable goal – even for our young colleagues. The diversity of rheumatological symptoms and the everyday 'chaos of rheumatology' have been structured and organized in this chapter using morphologically and pathophysiologically oriented reasoning.

Thereby, we take a strict *system of clinical reasoning*, reaching the diagnosis in steps or stages, without skipping any of the relevant steps or rushing to reach the finishing line (such as in the diagnosis of *Chlamydia*-induced *hemolytic anemia* and *pneumonia* in the *SLE* patient of CS 51, or prescription of MTX without a confirmed diagnosis in CS 28, or even the synovectomy in the case of suspected tumor from acute MTP 5 swelling with no *RF* and anti-*CCP*-Ab control, which shortly thereafter proved to be high, CS 14).

This integrated pathway appears to be more effective, and no more difficult, than the agreeable alternative in differential diagnosis, i.e., the careful *readout* of numerous diseases with known lead symptoms, e.g., *arthritis* and *myositis*.

To visualize the colorful, varied pattern of symptoms of *CTD* and/or *vasculitis*, the *following standardized steps* are recommended, which are also depicted in Rheumatology Tree 2 (See **RCS**, Chap. 1.4).

Step 1 Document the lead symptoms (nonspecific B symptoms).

The initial symptoms of these diseases are mostly entirely nonspecific (CS 25). They involve – primarily and fundamentally – *B symptoms* of unknown origin (Chap. 8) or mono-/oligosymptomatic connective tissue symptoms. Once they have been captured in detail, the next step should be taken and examined.

Step 2 Speculate on the systemic nature with a view to a potentially rheumatic disease.

The tricky part is to identify a systemic disease from the multitude of symptoms, or give a prognosis on the basis of mono symptoms. It is important thereby to be able to establish the *general criteria of a systemic disease*. Consideration must thus be given to the presence of:

- *Organ-/system* involvement of varying severities and combinations
- *B symptoms* (mostly varied)
- Such aspects are attributable to various diseases or conditions, in addition to *CTD* and *vasculitis*:
- *Oncological*
  - Lymphoproliferative
  - Metastatic
  - *Paraneoplastic* (can be manifested in the form of *CTD* and *vasculitis* or → Chap. 5)
  - *Tumors* of the kidneys, intestine and liver, which are difficult to diagnose (in early stages)
- *Infectiological* (which can also be associated with *CTD* and *vasculitis*)
  - *Sepsis, sepsis lenta* (secondary vasculitis)
  - *TB*
  - *Endocarditis*
  - *HIV*
  - *Syphilis*
- *Endocrinopathies*
  - *Hypothalamo-pituitary* syndrome
  - *Addison's*
- *Other diseases and conditions*
  - *Amyloidosis* (primary and secondary)
  - *Sarcoidosis*
  - Drug allergy and drug toxicity (e.g., *hypersensitivity vasculitis*)
  - Inflammatory bowel diseases (*Crohn's* disease, *Colitis ulcerosa*)
  - *Autoimmune hepatic and thyroid* diseases
  - Storage diseases (*Fabry's*, and *Gaucher's* diseases)

The systemic nature of such diseases has a different background to *CTD* and *vasculitis*. In these cases, it is basically a *localized process* (tumor, infection, hepatic or intestinal disease) which *is spreading* (metastases, TB, sepsis), or *incorporating*:

- The *connective tissue (paraneoplasias)*
- The *vascular system (secondary vasculitis* e.g., in *sepsis lenta*)
- The *immune system* (autoimmune diseases, *allergy, immune defects*)
- *Other diseases* that present with systemic symptoms (*lymphoproliferative, endocrinological, metabolic, sarcoidosis, amyloidosis*)

Once the diagnostic circle has been drawn in general terms, the next obligatory step can be taken.

Step 3 Oncological infectiological and other systemic diseases must be ruled out; cortisone-dependent diseases.

Before reflecting on such diseases, *priority must*, as a rule, be given to *CTD* and *vasculitis* (just as, in the same way, *peritonitis* must first be ruled out in any patient with abdominal pain), mainly on account of the extremely varied forms of therapy. *To think of this prevents a doctor's odyssey* a statement made with regard to *vasculitis*, and applying also to *CTD*.

Furthermore, only cases are considered in which none of the aforementioned, nonrheumatic diseases have been ascertained, and the *B symptoms* (particularly fever, CRP) as well as *organ involvement* (e.g., pulmonary infiltration) cannot be influenced by intensified antibiotic therapy. Subsequently – preferably once all other means of diagnosing a systemic rheumatic disease have been exhausted – cortisone therapy is initiated in order to check whether it is a cortisone-dependent disease.

Cortisone-dependent disease is a generic term for diseases responding to glucocorticoids, which, as the most potent anti-inflammatory substances, cannot be surpassed. They include many diseases in which the release of *pro-inflammatory cytokines* and *antibody-mediated reactions* are of pathogenetic relevance. Cortisone is administered, preferably at high doses, as pulse therapy (e.g., Decortin® 250–500 mg *IV* or Fortecortin® 8–6 mg *IM* or *per os* for 3–7 days) to ultimately investigate the presence of any inflammatory processes or others involving the release of pro-inflammatory cytokines. When applying such diagnostic procedures (*ex juvantibus* therapy) it should be noted that *this response* in some diseases is surprisingly *dose dependent*.

The most common *cortisone-dependent diseases* and *conditions* are:

- *CTD* and *vasculitis*, in the presence of exudative inflammation or activation of cytokine-producing cells, especially in the case of:
  - *Polymyalgia rheumatica*
  - *Vasculitis* of the large vessels (*giant-cell* and, in the early stage, *Takayasu's arteritis*)
  - *Vasculitis* of the small vessels (*Wegener's, Henoch-Schönlein* purpura, *cryoglobulinemic vasculitis, cutaneous leukocytoclastic vasculitis*)
  - *CNS* vasculitis
- All *autoimmune* antibody-mediated diseases or *conditions* (*hemolytic anemia, thrombocytopenia, exfoliative dermatitis*)
- All inflammatory *articular*, *spinal* and *STR* diseases (Sect. 1, Arthricular and Musculoskeletal Disorders)
- *Allergies*
- *Sarcoidosis* (systemic with organ involvement) or other granulomatous diseases
- *Ormond's* disease, particularly in the form of *periaortitis* and *periarteritis*
- Lymphoproliferative diseases (*lymphoma, leukemia*)
- *PCP*, *TB*, and *pneumonia*, wherein inflammatory components are strongly represented
- *Autoinflammatory diseases* and *syndrome* (Chap. 8.1)

This is by no means a complete list and does not allow for the presumption of *CTD* and/or *vasculitis* if cortisone elicits a response. *Lymphoproliferative* and other *immunological diseases*, for instance, will similarly show a response. Fortunately the diagnostic circle closes in a little due to this response to cortisone; however, the diagnostic problem is nowhere near resolved.

The concept of using a combination of antibiotics and cortisone as a trial therapy *(ex juvantibus)* causes greater confusion (and unfortunately cannot be avoided in difficult diagnostic cases, particularly in intensive medicine). If an improvement is achieved as a result, the *distinctions* between the infectiological and immunological diseases (the most common issue) remain just as unclear as before.

Conversely, if there is *no response to high-dose cortisone therapy*, a diagnosis of CTD and/or *vasculitis* is hardly likely as far as the *sclerotic, thrombotic, and necrotic* damage from such diseases is concerned. The seemingly inflammatory symptoms in the connective tissue and organs, such as in the case of *Fabry's* and *Gaucher's* disease (metabolic lysosomal *storage diseases* with arthritis, renal, cardiac, hepatic, blood, CNS involvement), could thus be distinguished from the inflammatory diseases. The same also applies, e.g., when investigating *elevated CK* or making a differential diagnosis of *myositis* or *myopathy*. If there is *no response to cortisone, florid myositis* (with the exception of *inclusion body myositis*) can, as a rule, be excluded.

It would be preferable to be able to prove the existence of *CTD* and/or *vasculitis* by other means than the response to cortisone (a number of clinical and immunological aspects of a *cortisone-dependent disease* can thereby be attenuated or lost).

Prior to administering cortisone, the nonspecific *B symptoms* should be considered from the viewpoint that perhaps *CTD* or *vasculitis* exists. Rapid *weight loss* and/or *fever* with chills are indicative primarily of *vasculitis* or highly active *SLE*. Well-tolerated *fever* is typical of active *SLE*, and *CRP* elevations with chills are not ruled out in the case of a true episode of *SLE* (Chap. 8.4), which, incidentally, will regress under high-dose cortisone therapy. Differential diagnostics with a view to whether *CTD, vasculitis, infection* (most common cause of death in *SLE*), or other diseases are present should be approached and considered step by step.

To differentiate between *inflammatory rheumatic diseases* and conditions involving *infection*, measurement of *procalcitonin* has been a recent development. An increased level is *almost* exclusively associated with *bacterial* (not without exceptions, e.g., *Legionella* infection), *parasitic* or *fungal infections*, but *not with viral infections*. Once the aforementioned distinctions have been made, as, e.g., in our case (CS 25, Fig. 112), a further diagnostic step, directed primarily at *CTD* or *vasculitis*, should be taken.

Step 4 Which connective tissue structures, organs (systems), and vessels are affected? Form the major syndromes. *Question themorphological diagnosis.*

The *clinical and morphological entirety* of these diseases should be regarded as a basis for confirming a diagnosis of *CTD* or *vasculitis*, requiring at the same time *methodical, broad, and in-depth* – in the same way that the connective tissue and vessels present themselves morphologically – *clinical examination*. From this point onwards, and possibly somewhat sooner, the *distinctions* between these diseases are important and can be achieved.

When interpreting the data obtained, two difficulties must be noted: on the one hand *the systemic nature* of a disease cannot be identified *(hypodiagnosis)* on account of

(a) Inadequate documentation of history
(b) Hidden symptoms
(c) Incomplete clinical and morphological tests
(d) Lack of adjustment when screening for system disease

On the other hand, such diseases are *wrongly diagnosed (hyperdiagnosis)* if a systemic nature *is identifiable*, but in fact does not exist in association with *CTD* or *vasculitis*, but rather with other diseases or conditions, e.g., *vasculitis* in *infections* or *allergies* (see above). To prevent false diagnosis, the major syndromes should first be formed – namely, the involvement of connective tissue structures and systems/organs (Chaps. 9 and 10) – and then checked through.

It must be remembered thereby that *connective tissue* and *multiorgan involvement* is on the one hand a *common characteristic* of *CTD* and/or *vasculitis*, while on the other hand the relevant symptoms with a view to their severity, combinations, and pathogenetic modifications are *highly individual and even unique in each patient.* In this respect, such *checks* should be *systematic* and *methodical*, by applying the motto, '*don't avoid anything*' or without omitting anything, and starting with the symptoms and history.

The symptoms help identify *the incorporation* of:

(a) *Connective tissue structures:*
   • Photodermatitis, "butterfly rash," induration → *skin*
   • Arthralgia, swelling, impaired mobility → *joints*
   • Myalgia, myasthenia → *muscles, fasciae*
   • Sattle-nose or swollen auricle → *cartilage*
(b) *Vascular system*:
   • Purpura, ulcerations of the skin and mucosa (aphthae)
   • *Claudicatio intermittens* (extremities and when chewing)
   • *Claudicatio arteriosa* ("no strength in the legs," CS 3)
   • Scalp pain, and *Claudication* of the jaw and tongue
   • Blue and/or white, or black fingers and toes, nail-fold necrosis, gangrene
   • Pain, numb sensations, motor deficits (mono/polyneuropathic symptoms)
   • Hemoptysis (alveolar hemorrhage)
   • Episcleritis and loss of vision
   • Sudden loss of hearing, bloody nasal secretion
   • Angina pectoris or myocardial infarction (history)
   • Abdominal pain and bloody feces (melena)
   • Thrombophlebitis and thrombangitis
(c) *System-/organ involvement:*
   • Dyspnea headache/chest pain, arterial hypertension, leg edema → *heart-lungs-kidneys*
   • Dysphagia → *esophagus*
   • Dry mouth and eyes → *salivary glands*

Without being nosologically specific (irrespective of *butterfly rash* in *SLE*, sclerodermic patches in *SSc*, marked muscular symptoms in *PM/DM*, open wounds in *panarteritis nodosa*, lack of pulse in *Takayasu's arteritis*), these carefully and systematically documented symptoms play a *pivotal role* in the further search for *CTD* or *vasculitis*.

When screening for *discriminatory symptoms*, such symptoms should be considered in correlation on account that they often overlap, and on account of their severity. If the above mentioned *vascular problems* predominate, for instance, perhaps in the form of *myalgia*, *arthralgia*, and *renal* and/or *pulmonary* involvement, thoughts should turn more to *primary vasculitis*. *Arthritis*, *scleroderma*, and *sicca* syndrome with *multiorgan involvement*, should initially be considered with a view to *CTD*. The specific questions addressed in clinical examinations should enable further differentiation.

The history should answer the following important questions:

(a) *The pattern of the actual condition* by documenting the nature of the connective tissue and multiorgan involvement

(b) *The individual nature of the emergence and progress* of diseases are *symbols of severity and prognosis*, which depend on genetically induced (auto)immune activities or the intensity of antigen stimulation, and are the major features of *CTD* (*SLE*, *SSc* and *PM/DM*) and certain types of *vasculitis* (*panarteritis nodosa*, *Wegener's*, *giant-cell arteritis*). A distinction is thereby made regarding:

With all of these mono symptoms, the development over the course of typical multiorgan involvement (kidneys, lungs, secondary vasculitis) is rather unlikely, although extremely severe lead symptoms (e.g., *anemia*, *thrombocytopenia*) cannot be ruled out.

- *Acute progression*: pinpointing *the day of the disease*, different systemic changes suddenly develop in each patient along with *typical multiorgan involvement* with increased activity *over a few months*. Well-being can be restored by intensified therapy, but relapses generally cannot be avoided and the prognosis appears serious.
- *Subacute progression* is much less aggressive: *the typical combination of syndromes* is detectable during the subsequent *2–3 years*; the prognosis is much more favorable and tends to depend on the quality of therapy.
- *Chronic progression* is minimally aggressive, with years of hidden mono-/oligo-symptoms, which are not necessarily typical of *CTD*.
- *Chronic SLE* has the following masks:
  - *Arthritis-pleuritis*
  - *Skin* changes (*LE*)
  - *Autoimmune thrombocytopenia* (*Werlhof* syndrome, CS 27)
  - *Autoimmune hemolytic anemia* (secondary, CS 51)
  - *Epileptic* episode (*CNS* vasculitis)
- Chronic *systemic sclerosis*:
  - *Raynaud's* syndrome
  - *CREST* syndrome (CS 32, 58)
  - *Localized scleroderma* (*circumscripta*)

- *PM/DM*
  - *Myasthenia*
  - *Muscular atrophy*
  - *Myalgia*
- *Panarteriitis nodosa/microscopic polyangiitis*
  - Selective *cutaneous ulceration*(s) /Fig. 2/
  - *Macular-nodular* skin changes (Fig. 33)
- *Wegener's* disease:
  - Chronic *sinusitis* (Fig. 86)
  - Chronic *mastoiditis*
  - *Sialadenitis*

(c) *Pattern of multiorgan involvement* over the course, namely, which systems and organs have already been affected, and the consequences.

(d) *Investigation of the causes* for the symptoms of *CTD* or *vasculitis* (*secondary diseases*)
  - *Drug-induced SLE* and *vasculitis* (*hypersensitivity vasculitis* or other /CS 42/)
  - *Chemically* induced *scleroderma* (silicon, polyvinyl chloride, *eosinophilia-myalgia* syndrome, impurity in the manufacture of L-tryptophan)
  - *Secondary CTD* and *vasculitis* arising from *paraneoplasia* (Chap. 5).

(e) *Administered therapy* in detail, its efficacy and tolerability.

(f) *Individual provocative factors*, e.g., para-allergic (medications, vaccinations, sun exposure), endocrine (pregnancy), and stress.

(g) *Concomitant diseases and conditions* (drug-induced, infections, immune defects).
Assessment of general health can be regarded as the *starting point for appropriate therapy* in terms of the selection of basic medications and their intensity.
Consideration must be given thereby to:
  - *B symptoms*, especially fever, weight loss
  - *Highly florid articular* or *vascular* symptoms (exudative *arthritis*, circulatory disorders)
  - *System* and/or *organ involvement* in all its breadth and severity
  - *Functional deficits* in the major organs (kidneys, lungs, heart, CNS)
  - *Complications*: secondary *infections*, *Cushing's* syndrome, surgical (*gangrene*).

When *grading* the *general health*, it is not always simple to decide whether the process is connected to an *episode* of a disease or to *drug-induced adverse effects* or – a third possibility – to *functional deficits*, e.g., renal insufficiency, as a result of *lupus nephritis* or hypertension in *SSc*.

The extreme generalization of activity in *SLE, SSc* (known as *hypertensive crisis*) or generalized *scleroderma* with pulmonary restriction, *renal failure, CNS*, and *pulmonary* involvement, *pulmonary hypertension* in *vasculitis*, is of particular significance. If nosological diagnosis can already be guaranteed at this point by immunological examinations (→ Step 8), which is good, the above mentioned problems are no less complicated.

Clinical examination is carried out with the aim of ascertaining *typical multiorgan involvement and degree of activity*, in order to be able to choose the correct *therapeutic strategy*. This is just as complex as the clinical and morphological patterns of *CTD* or *vasculitis*.

The *degree of activity* is measured from the *severity* of the following syndromes:

- *B symptoms*, primarily *fever* and *weight loss*
- *Organ* involvement: pneumonitis, nephritis, CNS vasculitis, Raynaud's syndrome
- *Connective tissue* involvement: polyarthritis, polyserositis, cytopenias for *SLE*, *MCTD*
- *Generalized scleroderma* (cutaneous induration) in *SSc*
- *Generalized myositis* of the transverse and smooth muscles in *PM/DM*
- *Sicca* syndrome in *Sjögren's* syndrome
- Severe and pronounced *circulatory disorders* with ischemia or necrosis in the end organs (heart, CNS, intestine) and distal extremities (*rat-bite necrosis, gangrene*) in all forms of *vasculitis*
- *Abdominal pain* in *panarteritis nodosa, Takayasu's arteritis, Henoch- Schönlein* purpura
- *Bronchial asthma* in *Churg-Strauss* syndrome
- *Loss of vision* or hearing in *SLE, Sjögren's* syndrome, *giant-cell arteritis, Cogan's, Wegener's, Behçet's* disease and other forms of *vasculitis*.

It is important thereby to establish the *dynamics of the activity and of organ-system involvement* during therapy, and monitor them closely.

Step 5 Dominant pathomorphological changes (inflammatory/ exudative or proliferative/ fibrotic or sclerotic/dystrophic). Questioning the *pathophysiological* diagnosis and *therapeutic objectives*.

The *morphological changes in the connective tissue* (with *CTD*), *vessels* (with *vasculitis*) and *internal organs* or *systems* (in both groups) develop in just as varied and progressive a way as the clinical course. Such changes have not *only similar*, but also *varying* and *discriminatory characteristics*, which can look entirely different in the event of an episode or when activity is minimal, as well as in a remission – as if two different diseases (in actual fact two sides to one disease) were to exist.

This applies perhaps to each disease in these two groups: initially, there are florid, highly inflammatory changes, behind which the *exudative components* of an inflammation are certainly concealed, requiring anti-inflammatory therapy – preferably with *glucocorticoids*. During and after therapy in particular, or quite spontaneously, these changes progress into the *proliferative* state, which tends to require alternative, i.e., *immunosuppressive therapy*. At this point, a colorful combination of *fibrotic and sclerotic* changes develops, which entails hardly any inflammation, with a *thrombotic and necrotic* process, which is able to induce irreversible end-organ damage.

Some diseases (*SSc, fibrotic fasciitis*, and *vasculitis* of the large vessels) entail, virtually from the start, proliferative and fibrotic changes. *Granulomatous* inflammation is typical for *sarcoidosis* (Figs. 83, 90), systemic *granulomatosis, Wegener's* (Figs. 86, 96, 112), changes in rheumatoid nodules in *RA* bone and pulmonary involvement (Figs. 36ab), and in the skin for *Granuloma annulare* and Churg-Strauss granuloma (in a similar way to rheumatoid nodules) and for *TB*.

At the same time, it is characteristic for such processes to start from the beginning at different locations. Thus, each patient is found to have a *unique combination* of different morphological changes.

Our task is to identify the *prevalent pattern of involvement* of the affected, clinically relevant target organs and systems, and proceed with the correct therapy.

Step 6 Pattern of connective tissue, organ-(system) and vascular symptoms form distinct syndromes. Questions: *Nosological entity, systemic or localized problems*

Once the other non-rheumatic diseases have been ruled out, the major syndromes (Chaps. 8, 9 and 10) defined in their extent and their severity, and their morphological background explained, the next question should be answered, namely, which *entity* is found, and whether it is perhaps an exceptional case whereby, e.g., with a chronic variant of *CTD* or *vasculitis*, there are merely local changes without involvement of an organ-/system (→Step 4). *The individual clinical picture*, as the target of each diagnostic process, is described well by the term *pattern of involvement*

The question of entity is linked to the *dominant syndromes and their combinations*. The most common associations thereby are:

- *Exudative connective tissue and organ symptoms*, associated with *SLE* and *MCTD: arthritis, dermatitis, polyserositis, glomerulonephritis*
- *Polychondritis relapsing* (Fig. 29)
- *Fibrotic-sclerotic symptoms* associated with *SSc, MCTD, fasciitis*:
  - Skin induration (*scleroderma, sclerodactyly*)
  - Peripheral circulatory disorders (*Raynaud's* syndrome, *osteolysis*)
  - *Pulmonary fibrosis*
- *Myalgia and myasthenia* are associated with *PM/DM, MCTD, SSc, vasculitis*
- *Sicca* symptoms are associated with *Sjogren's* syndrome or disease
- Recurrent *mucosal ulcerations* are associated with *Behcet's* disease (Fig. 76), *Wegener's, SLE* (CS 64).
- *Vascular symptoms* associated with *primary* or *secondary vasculitis* should, at this point, be documented in full and categorized according to vascular types.[13] Hereunder, there are a few clinical and morphological associations: *vasculitis* of the small and large vessels may affect medium-sized arteries, but *vasculitis* of the large and medium-sized vessels as a rule does not affect (with the exception, possibly, of *panarteritis nodosa)* the smaller vessels.
1. *Large vessels* (aorta and large or medium branches leading to the extremities or the head, and the kidneys), involving:

  - *Giant cell arteritis*, most common form of vasculitis in persons *over the age of 50 (the average age of onset is 72)*, possibly associated with *Polymyalgia rheumatica*, an inflammatory disease typical in persons *over the age of 65, rarely >50 years*
  - *Takayasu's arteritis* presents in the form of *stenoses* in the said arteries (Fig. 61) and ischemic organ damage, preferentially affects young women (CS 21)

- *Cogan* syndrome that primarily affects young adults is associated with ocular inflammation, audiovestibular dysfunction, and may take the form of aortitis
- *Behcet's* disease is one of the rare forms of vasculitis, also typically affecting the small- and medium-sized vessels, large arteries, and veins
- *Polychondritis relapsing* (Chaps. 3.11.6 and 11.8).

Clinical:

- *New onset of headache or temporal headache,* vertigo
- Shoulder pain and stiffness (in *polymyalgia rheumatica*)
- *Claudicatio intermittens* or provocable pain on exertion: walking, lifting the arms and chewing (*jaw claudication*); acute *claudicatio arteriosa* in thrombosis of the *aorta abdominalis* "no strength in the legs" (CS 3)
- *Leriche's* syndrome can present within the context of *aortoiliac disease* (See Chap. 9.2.5, Figs. 12, 132)
- *Visual disorders and blindness* (when other causes are ruled out)
- *Abnormal* temporal artery (pressure pain, swelling)
- *Fever* of unknown origin, *ESR*, and *CRP* elevations (Chap. 8.4)
- *Aortic arch* syndrome (Chap. 9.2.7, CS 21)
    - *Decreased* brachial artery pulse (to be checked in all extremities)
    - *Unequal* arm blood pressure of > 10 mm Hg between the arms
    - *Stenosis* (Fig. 61) and occlusion of the arteries in the extremities (Figs. 47, 113), and *A.renalis*
    - *A. subclavia* or aortic *bruit*
- *Hearing loss* and deafness
- *Arterial hypertension* (renal artery stenosis in *Takayasu's arteritis*)

2. *Medium-sized vessels* (visceral arterial trunks, e.g., of kidneys, heart, CNS, or mesenteric region). These are affected by *panarteritis nodosa* and *Kawasaki's* disease (mostly found in children), *primary CNS* vasculitis, and *Buerger's* disease , and secondary vasculitis in *RA* and *CTD*.

Clinical:

- *Infarctions* (*cerebral,* as in Fig. 17, *cardiac* /CS 21, 26/, renal, *intestinal* /CS 48/, extremities,* Fig. 47)
- The *medium and small vessels* are affected by the following symptoms:
    - *Myalgia* and muscular tenderness, *arthralgia* often without swelling, acute onset and severe
    - Palpable painful *nodes* along the length of the vessels (Fig. 33)
    - *Livedo racemosa and reticularis* (Figs. 2, 20a, 30–31)
    - Deep *cutaneous ulcerations* mostly of a necrotic-thrombotic nature (Figs. 2, 10–11, 30-31) and *CTD* (Fig. 71).
    - *Rheumatoid vasculitis* (Figs. 55, 101).
    - *Retinal artery occlusion* (Chap. 10.8.3)
    - *Mono-/polyneuropathic* syndrome (CS 48, 72), optic neuritis.
    - Audivestibular dysfunction (Chap. 10.9.3).
    - Monoclonal gammapathy with cryoglobulinemia (Fig. 132)
    - *Abdominal pain* in pseudoileus and renal vein thrombosis /CS 29/, intestinal necrosis (CS 48)
    - *Malabsorption* in intestinal ischemia and necrosis (CS 48)
    - Angina pectoris, *myocardial infarction* (CS 21, 26)

- *Testicular pain* (orchitis, hemorrhage, CS 12)
- Diastolic *arterial hypertension*
- *Hepatitis B* detection associated with *panarteritis nodosa*
- *Hepatitis C* associated with *cryoglobulinemic vasculitis* / Figs. 56ab/.

3. The predominantly *small vessels, small vessel vasculitis* (venoles, capillaries, arterioles, and intraparenchymal distal arterial system), involving:
   - *ANCA-associated vasculitis*
     - *Wegener's granulomatosis*
     - *Churg-Strauss* syndrome
     - *Microscopic polyangiitis*
     - *Drug-induced*
   - *Rheumatoid vasculitis* (Fig. 100)
   - Giant-cell arteriitis and IMIED
   - *Henoch-Schönlein* purpura
   - *Essential cryoglobulinemia* (Figs. 56ab)
   - *Hypersensitivity vasculitis*
   - *Behçet's* disease
   - *Urticarial vasculitis*
   - *Aortoiliac disease* (Fig. 132)

Clinical:
- Skin lesions (Chap. 9.1)
- Peripheral circulatory disorders
  - *Raynaud's* syndrome (Fig. 52)
  - *Ulcerations* (cutis - subcutis /Fig. 71/, mucosa /Fig.76/)
  - *Osteolysis* (Figs. 34, 54)
  - *Gangrene* (Fig. 47)
  - Alopecia areata (Fig. 82)
- *Mono-/polyneuropathy* (*peripheral nerve involvement*), Chap. 9.7
- Sudden *loss of hearing*, tinnitus, sinusitis, crusty-bloody rhinitis (*ENT involvement*), Chap. 10.9
- *(Epi)-Scleritis* /Fig. 57/ and visual affectation (*ocular involvement*), Chap. 10.8
- *Microhematuria*, proteinuria (*renal involvement*), Chap. 10.1
- *Hemoptoe* due to alveolar hemorrhage (*pulmonary involvement*), Chap. 10.2

The prevalent *connective tissue* and *multiorgan involvement* is most likely indicative of *CTD*. If the *vascular syndromes* are disproportionately pronounced, thought must be given to one of the many types of *vasculitis*. The next step should contribute largely to drawing a dividing line between *CTD* and *vasculitis* as well as differentiating amongst the relevant disease groups.

As far as the *distinctions* between *CTD* and *vasculitis* are concerned, the question of the actual primary involvement must be answered: if the *vessels* are affected, then which ones (in such a case consideration is to be given mostly to *primary vasculitis*)? Or if it is more of the *connective tissue*, then what is the morphological and pathophysiological nature (in this case, the concentration is mostly on *CTD*, possibly with *secondary vasculitis*)? It is essential here to rule out other diseases, especially tumors (Chap. 5), and ascertain relatively specific immunological activities (Chap. 11). Such associations are presented in Rheumatology Tree 2 (See **RCS**, Chap. 1.4)

As far as the *distinctions within one group of diseases* are concerned, a *pattern of involvement* must be identified. This comprises mainly the diagnostic criteria. For instance, if the numerous forms of *arthritis* and *myositis* can be differentiated on account of the specific pattern (see syndromes in Section 1 and 2). The *pattern of involvement* is also discernible from the more or less disease-specific constellations – *from individual syndromes to diseases* (Chap. 14.1) and *from combined syndromes to diseases* (Chap. 14.2), where further *diagnostic pathways* have also been explained.

Step 7 Association with tumors and other diseases.

Questions: *Causal diagnosis* and concomitant diseases or conditions

The close association of *CTD* and *vasculitis* with *tumors* is presented in Chap. 5. There is evidently a certain genetic burden in rheumatic diseases, e.g., *HLA-B27*-positive patients, or hereditary valvular heart defects in children of mothers with *SLE*, who demonstrate a particular immunological profile (*SS-A/Ro, SS-B/La*).

Another fact is that *CTD* and *vasculitis* are to be regarded more as introverted autoimmune diseases, but are not an exception in terms of pathology. They are triggered or even induced by certain external factors:

- *Sun* (ultraviolet) exposure for *SLE* (CS 38)
- *Medications* (hydralazine, minocycline, TNF-blockers) for *drug-induced SLE, hypersensitivity vasculitis* (CS 41, 42), *ANCA*-associated vasculitis
- *Silicon, polyvinyl chlorides* for *SSc* or *scleroderma*-type changes
- *Hepatitis B* antigenemia in *panarteritis nodosa*
- *Hepatitis C* and chronic hepatic diseases for *cryoglobulinemic vasculitis* (CS 20)
- *Stress*, possibly for all forms of *CTD* (the classic picture of acute systemic *scleroderma*, and above all *sclerodactyly* syndrome, painted by *Ivan Turgenev* in his story *Living Relic* (1867), is impressive)
- *Infection* for *Henoch-Schönlein* purpura and *cutaneous leukocytoclastic vasculitis*
- *Allergy*, possibly of unknown etiology.

Whatever the case, such problems should be very *actively* tackled.

Step 8 Investigation of clinical, immunological, and inflammatory activities.

Clinical activity is associated with the *actual state* of a disease and changes spontaneously over the course, particularly during therapy, which has to be adapted to the present activity.

The activity of a disease can be measured by:

- Severity of the *B symptoms* (Chap. 8), particularly CRP and weight loss
- Activity and scope of the connective tissue syndrome, especially *arthritis, dermatitis, myositis* (Chap. 9)
- Scope and severity of *system-/organ involvement* (Chap. 10).

Almost each disease has established and practice-oriented *activity criteria* (e.g., *DAS* 28 in *RA, PsA* score). An example is given using *SLE* to demonstrate how the calculation is made in systemic diseases.

The disease activity index for *SLE* (*systemic lupus erythematosus disease activity index – SLEDAI*) represents nine organs-systems potentially affected by *SLE*.[5] The syndromes most important to *SLE* activity are assessed, depending on clinical relevance, using different point scores (from 0 to 8). *SLEDAI* is the sum of the descriptors found during consultation or during the 10 preceding days. Mild to moderate disease is indicated by a *SLEDAI* score of *10* or *less*; higher activity is indicated by a score of *more than 10*.

Once the correct diagnosis has been made, the syndromes are marked with scores (in brackets) to give you the opportunity to measure the disease activity yourself. This was established for estimating the new option in CYC-resistant *SLE*, namely, *HAP*.3 At the same time, histological signs of activity in the kidneys were analysed semiquantitatively before (Fig. 92) and after (Fig. 93) therapy.

The same principle, with minimal deviations, also applies to *vasculitis* and the *Birmingham vasculitis activitys Score (BVAS)*, for example.[19] This index also documents *nine* organs-systems with potentially clinically relevant symptoms, though each such syndrome (rarely symptom) is assessed in the preceding four weeks with scores of 0–12, thus achieving a *maximum score* (total from the 9 sub-scores) of *63* and minimum score of *0*. Such activity scores are not only indispensable in academic work,[3] but also in everyday practice, since firstly the *persistence* of a high score is known to be associated with increased *lethality* and secondly such an activity score provides justification for *treatment escalation*.

Immunological activities are incorporated in *SLEDAI* (but not in *BVAS*), while they reflect the pathogenetic mechanisms of both disease groups and/or the inner milieu of diseases and thus represent the foundation for assessment of the *individual immune status*, including *genetic predisposition*, *specific diagnosis*, and *follow-up*.

From a clinical viewpoint, the following objectives of immunological tests are to be considered:

- *Specific diagnostics* for *CTD* and *vasculitis*, *APS*, and arthritis, associated with infections (Chap. 11)
- *RA* (*anti-CCP*-Ab)
- *Organ-/system-specific* antibodies to
  - Erythrocytes, thrombocytes
  - Musculature (striated and smooth), heart, kidneys, liver, parotid
- *Assessment of immunological activity* using the parameters of
- *B-cell activation*
  - *RF* and other non-organ-specific antibodies (*ANA, ENA* etc.)
  - Cryoglobulins
  - Antiphospholipid antibodies
  - Immune complexes
  - Complement consumption (C3, C4)
  - CD19 or CD20 (especially important with rituximab therapy)
  - Hypergammaglobulinemia
  - Immunoglobulins (IgG, IgA, IgM, IgE)
  - False-positive Wassermann reaction
- *T-cell activation*
  - Level of T-lymphocytes of various markings

- *T- and B-cell cooperation*
  - Number of immunoregulatory cells (T4, T8 and others)
- *Cytokine production:*
  - IL-2r
  - IL-6
- *Nonspecific resistance factors*
  - Complement
  - Phagocytosis
- *Immunomorphology*
  - Plasma lymphocytic infiltration in the muscles, internal organs, bone marrow (see below)
  - Immune complexes and immunoregulatory cells in the bioptates
  - LE phenomenon
- Determination of *genetic predisposition* and prognostic factors:
  - HLA-B27 (on suspicion of *SpA*)
  - HLA-DR4 (associated with rapid progression of *RA*)
  - HLA-B51 (if the course of *Behçet's* is severe).
- Current *immunological diagnostic methods* are mostly capable of distinguishing between *CTD* and *vasculitis* on account of the specific markings and associations See Chaps. 11.1 and 11.2.[12, 15, 21, 23] *The specific* immunological *markers* enable confirmation of the respective diagnosis in up to 40-100% of cases, depending on the entity and test method (Chap. 11).
- *Biochemical methods* are extremely helpful in the presence (or absence) of inflammation, as well as to specific diagnosis and follow-up.
- *Inflammatory parameters* (high values must always be investigated (Chap. 8.4)
  - *ESR*
    - Often selective (no CRP) increase in *CTD, polymyalgia rheumatica*
    - In *vasculitis* associated mostly with *CRP*
  - *CRP* (indispensable activity parameter)
    - Often *lacking* in even very active forms of *CTD*, except *SLE*
    - *Unexplained increase*, as *lead symptom*, often associated with *primary vasculitis (polymyalgia rheumatica, giant-cell* and *Takayasu's arteritis, panarteritis nodosa, undifferentiated vasculitis, polychondritis relapsing), Still's* disease
  - *Fibrinogen, alpha-2-gammaglobulins* (acute phase proteins).
- *Biochemical*, relatively disease-specific *parameters* in
  - *PM/DM*:
    - *CK* or *CK-MB* elevations (Chap. 9.6.4)
    - *Myoglobin* (in urine)
    - *LDH + GPT + GOT + aldolase*
  - *Hemolytic anemia* (Chap. 10.10.1)
  - Very high *ferritin* (*Still's* disease /associated with high level of *LDH + GPT + GOT* → CS 62, Fig. 131/, hemochromatosis /CS 50/, hemophagocytic syndrome → Chap. 10.10.5)
  - *Sarcoidosis* (serum *ACE* levels are often elevated /CS 33/ but up to 40% of patients with sarcoidosis have normal values as in this case /Fig. 83/ where the diagnosis was confirmed histologically).

Step 9 (Radio) morphological pattern of disease.

Investigation of *damage* caused by diseases

In *CTD* and *vasculitis*, such investigations are regarded as a diagnostic standard. *Radiological methods* (conventional X-ray, CT, DEXA, scintigram, angiogram, MRI, PET) are used for *confirmation of diagnosis and therapeutic monitoring* as well as for *estimation* of the *current activity or damage* arising during the course of a disease.

Radiological, sonography and other score methods are of relevance in the consideration of the following clinical situations:

- *Involvement of the heart, lungs, joints, parotid, eyes (pseudotumor)*, *CNS* and *muscles* (X-ray, sonography, CT, MRI)
- *Vascular* problems (which vessels, nature and extent of the changes) in *CTD* and *vasculitis* (MRI, CT, Doppler sonography, angiography, capillaroscopy, pulmonary function, pulmonary scintigraphy)
- Increased *fever*, *ESR*, *CRP* of unknown origin (Doppler sonography, angiography, CT, MRI, PET)
- *Presentation* of *myositis* (electromyography, MRI)
- *Complications from cortisone or basic therapy* and *concomitant diseases* (*osteoporosis*, gastrointestinal factors, *aseptic necrosis*)
- Investigations on suspicion of *paraneoplasia* (Chap. 13, Step 3).

Below are examples of the most important *radiomorphological syndromes* from our patients with *CTD* and *vasculitis* (see also Step 8 in Chap. 8):

- *CT* of the chest and other regions for investigating suspected tumor masses
  - *Rheumatoid nodules* in the lungs (Fig. 39, see also Figs. 36a and 38, X-ray chest)
  - Left *retrobulbar granuloma* in *Wegener's* disease (Fig. 96)
  - *Honeycomb lung, unexplained lymphadenopathy*, and *masses* (Fig. 79), in this case, with *histiocytosis X*
  - Causal investigation of *caverns* and *masses* (Fig. 112), in *Wegener's* in this case
  - *Pulmonary fibrosis* in *SSc* (Fig. 53), *MCTD* in this case with *tumor* (Fig. 85)
  - *Nephrocalcinosis* in *SLE* (Fig. 105)
- *MRI* for involvement of CNS-ENT and *Aorta abdominalis*
  - *ENT* involvement in *Wegener's* (Fig. 86)
  - *CNS multi-infarct* syndrome in primary *antiphospholipid* syndrome (Fig. 17, native)
  - *CNS* vasculitis (Fig. 50, with contrast)
  - Involvement of *Aorta abdominalis* and *A. iliaca* in *Takayasu's arteriitis* (Figs. 77ab).
- *PET* is used to ascertain whether the following structures are affected:
  - Large vessels (*aorta* and its branches, Figs. 74, 77a) for suspected *Takayasu's* and *giant-cell arteritis, Behçet's*
  - Small vessels (lungs)
  - Periaortic or retroperitoneal structures for suspected *Ormond's* disease
  - Exclusion of *lymphoma*

A negative result does not rule out such diseases or conditions.

- *Aortic angiography* is used routinely for the diagnosis of vascular involvement
  - *Acute thrombosis with aortic stenosis* in primary antiphospholipid syndrome (Fig. 12) or vasculitis (Fig. 132)
  - Suspected *Takayasu's arteritis* (Figs. 61, 77a, in this case MR angiography)

Chapter 14 describes the correlations between relevant radiological syndromes and diseases.

The (immuno) morphological examinations (Chap. 11.6) are indispensable and should be carried out as early as possible in order to enable early initiation of immunosuppression and improvement of the prognosis. These examinations are performed predominantly on the following regions, while concentrating on the following issues:

- *Renal* biopsy (treatment-resistant *nephrotic* syndrome in *SLE, vasculitis*)
- *Muscle-skin* biopsy (diagnostic criterion for *panarteritis nodosa*)
  - *SLE* (*lupus band test:* mononuclear infiltration and band-shaped deposits of Ig and complement on the dermal-epidermal border lamella */junction/* also in skin changes that are not visible)
  - *SSc* (excessive accumulation of collagen in the skin and vessels)
  - *PM/DM* (in open muscle biopsy, perivascular and interstitial mononuclear infiltrates, muscle fiber necrosis, muscular atrophy, and fibrosis are visible)
  - *Sjögren's* syndrome (lymphoplasmocytic infiltrates, defined by focus score)
  - *Wegener's* disease (*necrotic vasculitis* of the small to medium vessels in the kidneys */glomerulonephritis/* and other organs or systems, for example: cutaneous extravascular necrotizing granuloma, so-called "Churg-Strauss granuloma"; *granulomatous inflammation* may appear *without vasculitis*)
  - *Churg-Strauss* syndrome (eosinophilic and granulomatous inflammation, *necrotic vasculitis* of the small to medium vessels, known as allergic granulomatosis), "Churg-Strauss granuloma"
  - *Giant cell* and *Takayasu's arteritis* (*giant-cell, media-necrotizing granulomas* and lymphoplasmocytic infiltrates, mostly *A. temporalis* in *giant cell arteritis*)
  - *Panarteritis nodosa* (in the medium-sized arteries: *granulocytic infiltration* of the wall, microaneurysms, stenoses, necroses, thrombosis, also on angiography of the mesenteric vessels)
  - *Microscopic polyangiitis* (*necrotizing* vasculitis of the capillaries, venoles or arterioles; in all cases, the small and medium vessels in the kidneys could also be affected)
  - *Cryoglobulinemic vasculitis* (*necrotizing leukocytoclastic vasculitis* of the small vessels, a type of *small vessel vasculitis*)
  - *Hypersensitivity vasculitis, small vessel vasculitis,* (*leukocytoclastic vasculitis* of the capillaries, venoles, arterioles; as a rule, only affecting the skin with lesions in the same stage, systemic signs spared or very rare)
  - *Urticaria vasculitis* targets the capillaries and postcapillary venules in the skin, mediated at least partially by immune complex deposition of IgG and C3 leading to the *leukocytoclastic destruction* of capillary walls
  - *Henoch-Schönlein* purpura *'small vessel vasculitis'* (*leukocytoclastic necrotizing vasculitis* of the small vessels /see above/ with *IgA* deposits in the skin of the extremities, renal glomeruli and gastrointestinal tract)

- *Buerger's* disease, also called *thromboangiitis obliterans* of the medium-sized arteries at the levels of the ankle and wrist, and superficial thrombophlebitis without evidence of internal organ involvement
- *Behçet's* disease typically affects the small-and medium-sized vessels, capable of also affecting large arteries, involving veins and causing venous thrombosis.
- *Primary vasculitis of the CNS*, limited to the brain and less commonly spinal cord, affects chiefly small and of medium-sized arteries; thrombosis and rupture can lead to infarction and hemorrhage of the surrounding tissue
- *Neuromuscular* biopsy (*N. suralis, M. trizeps surae*) for suspected *vasculitis* and *mono/ polyneuropathy, myositis, fasciitis*
- *ENT* biopsy for suspected *Wegener's* or other disease
- *Parotid gland* for suspected *Sjögren's* disease or *lymphoma* (following ultrasound and scintigram)
- *A. temporalis* (for suspected *giant-cell arteritis* following Doppler sonography)
- *All masses* (liver, lungs, kidneys, and parotid) to rule out *neoplasia*

It is particularly important to determine the *pathomorphology* of the processes (preferably from the affected areas and *before* immunosuppressive *treatment*), namely, whether there is any *granulomatous, necrotic, leukocytoclastic, sclerotic and proliferative* inflammation. Such data should be reconciled with the clinical findings. The clinical interpretation of some of these methods in our patients is presented in Chap. 11.6.

It is *clinically relevant*, when considering the entire clinical picture, to *separately grasp* the components of *activity and damage*, namely, the interaction between *current activity* and the *damage having taken place*, i.e., traces of scars from previous episodes and therapies. With such an approach, priorities must be very clearly identified – namely, what actually prevails in the given case: the *activity* of the disease, which is currently active and assailable; or the *damage*, which is to be treated, if at all, by other means; or the *harm* caused by the ongoing or completed *therapy*, which could be more harmful than the disease itself? Or is it a combination of all of them, as is often the case, and if so what is the logical sequence?

To estimate the *damage* from rheumatic diseases: attention is paid to *irreversible changes* (a period *covering 6 months* has been set for *SLE*) with no correlation to active inflammation and already apparent adverse effects of therapy (e.g., *diabetes mellitus, cataracts* from cortisone therapy or *pulmonary fibrosis* from MTX).

As concerns *articular* and *spinal* diseases, such damage is mostly ascertained *radiologically*, e.g., in *fibrosing/ankylosing arthritis* (Chap. 1.3.3) or *bamboo spine* with *syndesmophytes* and/or *spinal curvatures* in *AS* (Chaps. 2.2 and 2.5). In some common diseases (*RA, OA*, and *PsA*) or conditions (*sacroiliitis*), damage has been quantified by *stage* (mostly 3–4). These late sequelae of an inflammation do not rule out any presently existing inflammation. There is also a considerable discrepancy between the morphological (*stage*) and clinical (*pain*) picture of a disease. Hence, not every patient with a radiologically "broken" knee necessarily requires surgery. In such cases, the clinical indications should be given precedence. Further diagnostics and therapy should be deduced from such considerations.

In the case of *CTD* and *vasculitis*, such *damage* may be a remnant of prior activities affecting every organ or system, without exception. Some of this damage, in the form of *scarring*, must be clearly defined (e.g., in Figs. 32 and 101b) or, e.g., could result from *insult, myocardial infarction* or *lungs fibrosis*, long-term *neurological deficits, blindness, deaf,* etc. In *SLE*, such changes, regardless of their etiology, must be summarized and quantified, in fact, in a *damage index (SLICC/ACR,*[6]*),* if they have existed for at least 6 *months.* Identical *stable* damage from *vasculitis* has been documented by the *vasculitis damage index.*[11] What has become evident is that these two scores should be measured at least every six months/annually over the course of the disease in order to estimate the *extent* of the *damage* (the higher the total score, the greater the damage) and the *progression* of the disease (from an increase in the score over a certain period of time).

If the *timing of the damage,* particularly with renal, pulmonary or CNS insufficiency, cannot be clearly ascertained, it should be assumed that a *combination of activity and scarring* is present at the same time. The question of the relationship, in whichever form, can only be resolved over the course by means of *trial therapy,* e.g., with cortisone (for *CNS* symptoms) or immunosuppression (in *SLE* and *vasculitis*).

The degree of response to such therapy is to be interpreted as the presence, or even an indirect indication, of an inflammatory component or disease activity.

Such problems are also interpreted *morphologically* in essential renal involvement, whereby the prognostically relevant assessment of the *degree of activity and chronification* in the renal bioptates can be analysed successively. During effective therapy, in our case with high-dose azathioprine pulse therapy in CYC-resistant patients with *SLE* and *Wegener's,* the *activity index* dropped considerably,[3] albeit in line with the reduction in *renal insufficiency and proteinuria.* Whatever the case, such problems should be tackled using the *signs of activity and damage* from each rheumatic disease, investigated separately and accounted for in the formulation of the diagnosis.

Step 10 Preliminary diagnosis and consistency with known diagnostic criteria.

Central to the diagnosis of *CTD* and *vasculitis* are the syndromes, which embody the anatomical, or pathomorphological, and pathogenetic *similarities* of these diseases at the same time as the *peculiarities* of each one, and should be divided into four large subgroups (cf. Rheumatology Tree 2, → *RCS*, Chap. 1.4):

- *Connective tissue* syndrome
- *System-/organ* syndrome
- *Autoimmune* syndrome
- *Concomitant syndromes*

Once the other diseases have been ruled out (→ Steps 1–3), and clarification obtained for the *morphological substrate* of a disease with the *characteristics of connective tissue* and *system-organ damage* (→ Steps 4, 5, 6 and 8) in *association with the immunological and inflammatory activities* (→ Step 7), as well as the *causal problems,* all the requirements for ascertaining a certain diagnosis have been fulfilled.

"The *underlying disease must be the primary diagnosis.* The present manifestation is given as a *secondary diagnosis* provided it poses an independent and important problem in medical care".[17]

In our opinion, the *certain diagnosis* of *CTD* and *vasculitis* could only be achieved on account of the *aforementioned clinical, morphological, and immunological manifestations* and/or established syndromes. Such syndromes are ascertained and confirmed *according to priority* using differential diagnostic criteria at the first sign of a clinical situation.

These disease-specific syndromes also appear in the diagnostic criteria of a disease. Consequently, only at this stage can the *established, pivotal syndromes* be *compared* against the *known diagnostic criteria* of one or more diseases in order to be able to progress from *preliminary* diagnosis to *certain diagnosis of an underlying disease.*

The diagnosis is *confirmed* by making a *comparison* against the accepted diagnostic criteria for diseases or syndromes.

Step 11 Diagnostic formulation

The ultimate outcome of our considerations should comprise *all aspects of an underlying disease* or *condition* that are of pivotal importance to *individual therapy and prognosis.* Hence the detailed diagnostic formulation covers:

1. The *underlying disease as primary diagnosis (entity)*
2. The important *organ manifestations* or *syndromes* (by priority)
3. The important *connective tissue manifestations* or syndromes (by priority) as a *secondary diagnosis*
4. *Concomitant diseases* and syndromes (according to the guidelines for clinical practice. In: Coding Guidelines of Rheumatology, 2010[17])

Furthermore, the aspects relevant to *therapeutic scheduling and prognosis* (see above) are considered and to a large extent incorporated in the diagnostic formulation:

5. *The present activity* (highly active, moderate, minimal, remission)
6. *Immunological marking, morphologically and MRI-confirmed changes*
7. *Potential etiology* (e.g., *drug-induced SLE, SSc, vasculitis*)
8. *Onset* over time (acute, subacute, or chronic) and the *progressive nature* (progressive, stable, regressive) defined at the time of examination
9. If necessary, *status post intervention* (biopsies or surgery)
10. *Present therapy and condition* after completion of therapeutic measures

The diagnostic screening program for *CTD* and *vasculitis* has more *similarities* than differences to the *arthrological* screening program (Chap. 6). These common morphological, pathophysiological, causal and broad internal medical factors are at the same time the basis for the *integrated diagnostic program in each clinical discipline* (*RCS*, Chap. 1.1.1).

The *features/or peculiarities or distinctions* in the diagnosis of arthrological and systemic rheumatic diseases are of tremendous clinical relevance, however:

1. In *CTD* and *vasculitis*, there are *relatively few disease-specific syndromes:* of the *40* pathognomonic figures marked in Chaps. 2, 3 and the Appendix (all in *RCS*) with (*C*), only six are attributable to *CTD* and *vasculitis*. All other disease-specific figures in this book are arthrological diseases. The depicted syndromes in the patients with *CTD* and *vasculitis* are for the most part *not specific to a disease* (subgroup *B*) or *to a condition,* i.e., *they reflect only one morphological diagnosis* (subgroup *A*).

2. Consequently, in the case of connective tissue-/organ symptoms, *each syndrome initially should be regarded as a condition, rather than as an entity*, which would fit several diseases, e.g., *myocardial infarction* in a young woman with *Takayasu's arteritis* (CS 21) or a 73-year-old woman with *Behçet's* disease (CS 26).
3. No other group of diseases, with its syndromes, comes so close to *infections, tumors*, and other *systemic diseases* as do *CTD* and *vasculitis*, especially as far as the onset of a typical clinical pattern and the course is concerned. *Thinking about this as early as possible* is of pivotal diagnostic importance.
4. In the case of *secondary vasculitis, extra-articular manifestations* and to some extent similar (ANA, dsDNA, rheumatoid factors, etc) or absent *immunological activity*, there are *several transitional forms* and *vague distinctions* between individual forms of *CTD, vasculitis* and, e.g., *RA* or *SpA* with systemic symptoms, which can complicate nosological diagnosis.

The structured reasoning detailed in this chapter enables such diagnostic difficulties to be graded and categorized.

Algorithms for Connective Tissue Disease and Vasculitis

14

14.1
From Individual Syndromes to Diseases

(See Chap. 7 for Articular and Muskuloskeletal Disorders)

Here the simple diagnostic pathway is summarized, while considering the systemic diseases. A starting point is the recognition of the lead symptoms and syndromes which, individually, do not yet permit nosological classification but do encompass the entities that are to be taken into account. The list covers pivotal and discriminatory syndromes in stable combination, and potential diseases, which may pinpoint the further *diagnostic options* that still need to be *investigated* (Table 14.1).

14.2
From Combined Syndromes to Diseases

Here the simple diagnostic pathway is summarized, while considering the systemic diseases. A starting point is the recognition of the lead symptoms and syndromes which, individually, do not yet permit nosological classification but do encompass the entities which are to be taken into account. The list covers pivotal and discriminatory syndromes in stable combination, and potential diseases which may pinpoint the further *diagnostic options* which still need to be *investigated* (Table 14.2).

E. Benenson, *Rheumatology*, Symptoms and Syndromes
DOI: 10.1007/978-1-84996-462-3_14, © Springer-Verlag London Limited 2011

Table 14.1 Diagnostic pathways from leading syndromes to disease(s)

Syndromes	Diseases	Investigations
Puffy hands, symmetrical/Figs. 7, 66, 130c/	CTD* (MCTD), V**, allergy, angioedema	System-/organ involvement, CTD and V serology
Puffy hands, asymmetrical/Fig. 115/	Sudeck's syndrome, arthritis, septic	Traumas, surgery, lab (CRP), MRI
Contractures with calcinates, sclerodactyly/ Fig. 18/	SSc, CREST syndrome	System-/organ involvement, ANA, ENA
Contractures all fingers/Figs. 19, 43, 130a/	Arthropathy, RA, arthrosis (OA)	Neurological, RA/OA diagnostics
Contractures individual fingers/Figs. 63, 95/	RA, SSc, fasciitis, tumor, Dupuytren's contracture, also idiopathic	RA, SSc diagnostics, tumor screening, possibly MRI (poss. before surgery)
Deep ulcerations/Figs. 2, 10–11, 14, 30–31, 55, 71, 101a, 132/	Vasculitis, arterio-sclerosis obliterans, primary or secondary APS	CTD,V, RA, APS serology, biopsy, capillaroscopy
Aorta abdominalis stenosis, Leriche syndrome, aortoiliac disease/Figs. 12, 132/	APS with aortic thrombosis, Arteriosclerosis, V	CTD, V, APS serology, system-/organ involvement
CNS multi-infarct syndrome/Fig. 17/and diffuse nodules/Fig. 50/	APS, CNS-V, embolisms, arteriosclerosis	APS, CTD and V serology, system-/ organ involvement, rule out Foramen ovale
Livedo reticularis or racemosa/Figs. 2, 20a, 30–31/	CTD, V, borreliosis, APS	CTD, V, APS, borreliosis serology
Panniculitis/Figs. 6, 27, 71/	SLE, MCTD, erysipelas, ReA, phlegmona	CTD, ReA (Yersinia) serology; puncture, bacteriology
Erythema with subcutaneous nodes/Fig. 33/, *Erythema nodosum*/Fig. 109/	MPA, sarcoidosis, infectious condition	ANCA, biopsy, chest X-ray, Yersinia antibodies

* CTD- connective tissue diseases,
**V – vasculitis, for further abbreviations see index

Circular shadows with caverns/Figs. 38, 39, 112/ or with cysts/Fig. 79/or no caverns/Figs. 36a, 39, 85/	TB, tumors, WG, pneumonia, rheumatoid nodules, histiocytosis X	Exclusion diagnosis of such diseases as far as biopsy and surgery
Digital gangrene and rat-bite necrosis/Figs. 47, 113/	CTD, V, APS, arteriosclerosis obliterans, paraneoplasia	Organ involvement, ENA, ANCA, tumor screening, capillaroscopy
Raynaud's phenomenon/Figs. 16, 47, 52, 130c/	Primary and secondary (CTD, V)	System-/organ involvement, ANA, ENA, ANCA
Lung X-ray: diffuse milky changes/Fig. 53/	Pneumonia and alveolitis in SSc, MCTD, SLE, PM, sarcoidosis	System-/organ involvement, ANA, ENA, ANCA, ACE, diffusion capacity (DLCO)
Pulmonary (basal) sclerosis with or without hilar lymphadenopathy/Figs. 79, 91/	SSc, MCTD, PM, sarcoidosis, COLD, histiocytosis X	System-/organ involvement, ANA, ANCA, ACE
Palpable erythema/Figs. 56ab/	V, primary and secondary	V immunology, cryo V, exclusion of allergy, infec-tions, neoplasia
(Epi)-Scleritis/Fig. 57/	V, SpA, ReA, RA, idiopathic	Organ involvement, HLA-B27, immunology
Auricular chondritis (Fig. 29), symmetrical, spares the earlobe	Polychondritis relapsing	Organ involvement, exclusion of V, CTD, or myelodysplastic syndrome
A. subclavia stenosis/Fig. 61/	TA	Organ involvement and TA activity
Non-erosive arthritis with hand deformities/ Figs. 70, 72/	MCTD, SLE, polychondritis relapsing	ANA, ENA, hand X-ray, organ involvement
Enhancements in aorta on PET/Figs. 74, 77b/	TA	Organ involvement and TA activity
Pulmonary infiltrates/Figs. 36a, 38, 39, 75, 85/	Pneumonia, WG, MPA, neoplasia,	Exclusion diagnosis for such diseases

(continued)

Table 14.1 (continued)

Syndromes	Diseases	Investigations
Mucosal aphthae (mouth)/Fig. 76/	All CTD, MB, WG, MTX therapy	System-/organ involvement, immunology, genetics
Irregularities in aorta and *A. iliaca* on MRI angiography/Fig. 77a/	TA Aorta abdominalis	Rule out involvement of other arteries
Thrombocytopenic purpura/Fig. 78/	Idiopathic or secondary thrombocytopenia	Rule out SLE, system-/organ involvement, ANA, ENA, platelet antibodies
Alopecia areata/Fig. 82/	Secondary (SLE, SSc) and primary (skin disease)	Organ involvement, ANA, ENA, possible consultation (dermatology)
Callosities on the skin/Fig. 83/	Sarcoidosis, lymphoma, granuloma annulare	Skin biopsy, ACE, lung X-ray
Sinus masses/Fig. 86/	Sinusitis, WG, lymphoma, tumor	Biopsy, organ involvement, ANCA
Focal erythema, diffuse/Fig. 90/	Sarcoidosis, lymphoma, granuloma annulare	Biopsy, ACE, chest X-ray, system-/organ involvement
Periorbital edema with erythema/Fig. 94/	DM, idiopathic, paraneoplastic	System-/organ involvement, tumor screening
Pararorbital destruction/Fig. 96/	Tumor, WG, lymphoma	Biopsy, ANCA, system-/organ involvement
Palmar erythema and reddened finger tips/ Fig. 100/	Secondary V (in RA, neoplasias)	Broad immunology, tumor screening
Ulcus cruris/Figs. 55, 101 a/	Secondary V, venous thrombosis, Granuloma gangraenescens	System-/organ involvement, RA, V immunology, poss. biopsy
Several scars/Fig. 101b/	Status post effective therapy for *ulcus cruris*	History (see comments on Fig. 101)

Nephrocalcinosis/Fig. 105/	Sjögren's syndrome SLE, hyperparathyroidism	System-/organ involvement, tubular damage
'Butterfly erythema' 'saddle nose' deformity (refer to other textbooks),	SLE, LE, drug-induced SLE, WG, relapsing Polychondritis, cocaine abuse, congenital syphilis, midline granuloma, NHL, leprosy	System-/organ involvement, poss. drug-related
Swallowing difficulties, dysphagia/CS 58/	Tumor, CREST syndrome, fibromyalgia, esophagitis	Tumor screening, system-/organ involvement, tender points, CTD serology
Sicca syndrome and parotid enlargement /CS 56/	Sjögren's syndrome, primary and secondary, lymphoma/Chap. 10.7/	ANA, ENA, system-/organ involvement, poss. infection, medication, biopsy
Mono-/polyneuropathy/CS 18, 48, 72/	MS, CTD/MCTD, Sjögren's syndrome/and V/ CSS, PAN/	ANA, ENA, system-/organ involvement, neurological consult
Lymphadenopathy/CS 49, 59, 66/	CTD, Still's, lymphoma, metastasis	ANA, ENA, system-/organ involvement, biopsy
Coombs positive/CS 38/and aemolytic anemia/CS 51/	SLE or idiopathic	ANA, ENA, system-/organ involvement, biopsy
High rheumatoid factors with anti-CCP-Ab/CS 1, 10, 14, 68/	RA Felty's syndrome	RA diagnostics
High rheumatoid factors with no anti-CCP-Ab /CS 20, 53, 56, 70/	Cryoglobulinemia, Sjögren's syndrome, RA, autoimmune hepatitis, WG, CSS	ANA, ENA, ANCA, system-/organ involvement, proof of cryoglobulins
High ANA titers with no differentiation/CS 3 with dsDNA-Ab, not confirmed by Crithidia test, CS 16, 38/	MCTD, APS, autoimmune thyroiditis	ANA, ENA, system-/organ involvement, ACLA
ANA with dsDNA-Ab, confirmed by Crithidia test/RIA prior to therapy/CS 27, 29, 34, 51, 71/	SLE, not drug-related	ANA, ENA, system-/organ involvement

(continued)

Table 14.1 (continued)

Syndromes	Diseases	Investigations
ANA, SS-A and SS-B/CS 18, 49, 53, 56/	Sjögren's syndrome poss. with lymphoma	ANA, ENA, system-/organ involvement, biopsy
ANA with anti-Cemp-Ab (CS 32, 58)	CREST syndrome, SSc	ANA, ENA, system-/organ involvement
ANA with anti-RNP-Ab/CS 2, 24/	MCTD, SSc	ANA, ENA, system-/organ involvement
ANA with anti-Scl-70-Ab /CS 19, 54/	SSc, MCTD	ANA, ENA, system-/organ involvement
High liver enzymes and LDH /CS 62, 66/	Still's, tumors, hepatitis	Tumor screening, cortisone (prior to liver biopsy)
High cANCA/CS 48, 72, 73/	ANCA positive V, neoplasia	System-/organ involvement, ANCA, tumor screening
Elevated serum calcium/CS 56, 67/	Paraneoplasia, hyperparathyroidism	Hospital referral, tumor screening, parathormone
CK elevated/CS 54/	PM/DM, myopathy Hypo-/hyperthyroidism, sport activities (prior to examination)	ANA, ENA, system-/organ involvement, repetition, poss. Cortisone therapy
Hypereosinophilia/CS 72/	CSS, hypereosinophilia syndrome	ANCA, system-/organ involvement
Stable cytopenia or neutropenia in immunosuppressed RA patient/CS 68/	Myelodysplasia or myelotoxicity (immunosuppression), Felty's syndrome, SLE, T-cell leukemia	System-/organ involvement, bone marrow cytology, immunology (with neutrophil antibodies)
Ferritin increase in arthritis/CS 50/	Hemochromatosis, Still's	Hepatic, articular involvement
Sudden hearing loss and deafness, Sensorineurale syndrome	WG, Cogan's, Muckle–Wells syndrome, autoimmune sensorineurale sensorineurale hearing loss	System-/organ (eye, aorta) involvement, ANA, ANCA

Table 14.2 Diagnostic pathways from combined syndromes to diseases

Connective tissue syndrome with system-/organ involvement/Chaps. 9–10/	CTD and V, also undifferentiated, Gaucher's, Fabry's	CTD and V serology, system-/organ involvement
Response to cortisone/CS 18, 51, 62, 71 → Chap. 13.3/	Cortisone-dependent diseases: CTD, V, sarcoidosis, lymphoma and others	Response is no proof of inflammatory-rheumatic disease
Fever of unknown origin, CRP and ESR elevation/CS 25, 60, 62 → Chap. 8/	CTD (SLE, MCTD, CREST) and V (TA), Still's, septic form of Yersinia-associated arthritis	CTD and V serology, system-/organ involvement
Deterioration in general health with dramatic weight loss/CS 25, 48, 58/	V (with intestinal involvement), TA, Still's, CREST syndrome	CTD and V serology, system-/organ involvement, MRI-PET of aorta
Arthralgia, myalgia, fatigue, depression poss. with lymphadenopathy/CS 59/	Lymphoma, CTD, V, fibromyalgia, Gaucher's	CTD and V serology, system-/organ involvement (lymph nodes!), CRP
Myalgia, myasthenia, CK and TSH elevation/CS 54/	Myositis, PM/DM, hypothyroidism	Tumor screening, statins? Hypothyroidism
Myocardial infarctions in patients with no risk factors and poss. elevated CRP/CS 21, 26/	Coronaritis in TA, SLE, MB	ANA, ENA, system-/organ involvement
Exudative pleuritis with Raynaud's syndrome, lymphadenopathy, fever/CS 19, 38, 49/	Initial syndrome in SSc, SLE, Sjögren's syndrome, Still's, tumor	Tumor screening, CTD and V serology, system-/organ involvement, poss. cortisone administration
Polyserositis with CRP elevation/CS 62/	Still's, tumors	As with exudative pleuritis (see above)
Panmyocarditis or its sequelae/CS 24/	CTD (SLE, MCTD), rheumatic fever, borreliosis	Cardiological examination, cortisone, basic therapy
Autoimmune hepatitis	Primary or associated with SLE, SSc, sarcoidosis	ANA, ENA, system-/organ involvement, liver biopsy
Nephritis with renal hypertension and other syndromes	CTD (SSc, SLE) and V (PAN, Goodpasture syndrome)	ANA, ENA, system-/organ involvement, renal biopsy
Nephritis with nephrotic syndrome/Fig. 92, CS 34, 38, 71/	SLE, PM, MCTD,	ANA, ENA, system-/organ involvement, renal biopsy essential

References

1. Adabajo A, ed. *ABC of Rheumatology (ABC Series)*. Paperback: Wiley-Blackwell; 2009.
2. Benenson E. A program of diagnostic scrutiny in diffuse connective tissue diseases. *Klin Revmatologiia (Mosk)*. 1998;1:12-16 [Russian].
3. Benenson E, Fries JW, Heilig B, et al. High-dose azathioprine pulse therapy as a new treatment option in patients with active Wegener's granulomatosis and lupus nephritis refractory or intolerant to cyclophosphamide. *Clin Rheumatol*. 2005;24:251-257.
4. Benenson E, Blank H, Pelzer R et al. Magnetic resonance imaging (MRI)-confirmed soft tissue disorders as "model" for anti-inflammatory effect of LLLT (785 mm). Proceedings of the 6th International Congress of the World Association of Laser Therapy. Limassol (Cyprus), October 25–28, 2006; Medimond:63–67.
5. Bombardier C, Gladman DD, Urowitz MB, et al. Derivation of the SLEDAI. *Arthritis Rheum*. 1992;35:630-640.
6. Gladman D, Ginzier E, Goldsmith C, et al. The development and initial evaluation of the Systemic Lupus International Collaborating Clinics/American College of Rheumatology damage index for systemic lupus erythematosus. *Arthritis Rheum*. 1996;39:363-369.
7. Dzau VJ, Creaber MA. Diseases of the aorta. In: Wilson JD, Braunwald E, eds. *Harrison's Principles of Internal Medicine*. 12th ed. New York: McGraw-Hill; 1991. 1018.
8. Dougados M, van der Linden S, Juhlin R, et al. The European Spondylarthropathy Study Group: preliminary criteria for the classification of spondylarthropathy. *Arthritis Rheum*. 1991;34:1218-1227.
9. Hegglin R. *Differential Diagnosis Intrinsing Diseases*. Georg Thieme Verlag; 1961 [German].
10. Engert D, Bohlen H, Tesch H, Benenson E. Pains of the joints. In: Classen M, Diehl V, Kochsiek M, et al., eds. *Differential Diagnosis. Internal Medicine*. Munich/Vienna/Baltimore: Urban & Schwarzenberg; 1998:541-565.
11. Exley AR, Bacon PA, Lugmani RA, et al. Development and initial validation of the vasculitis damage index for the standardized clinical assessment of damage in the systemic vasculitides. *Arthritis Rheum*. 1997;40:371-380.
12. Imboden JB, Hellmann DB, Stone JH. *Current Rheumatology Diagnosis and Treatment*. 2nd ed. New York: Lange Medical Books/McGraw-Hill; 2007.
13. Jennette JC, Falk RJ, Andrassy K, et al. Nomenclature of systemic vasculitis. *Arthritis Rheum*. 1994;37:187-192.
14. Firestein CS, Budd RC, et al. *Kelley's Textbook of Rheumatology, Eighth Editions. Volume I and II*. Philadelphia: W.B. Saunders; 2009.
15. Klippel JH, Stone JH, Crofford LE, White HP, eds. *Primer on the Rheumatic Diseases*. 13th ed. Springer Science+Business Media; 2008

16. Klemperer P, Pollack AD, Baehr G. Landmark article May 23, 1942: diffuse collagen disease. Acute disseminated lupus erythematosus and diffuse scleroderma. *JAMA*. 1984;25: 1593-1594.

17. Coding Guidelines of Rheumatology, Version 2010 [German].

18. Kurmanalieva AK, Benenson E, Mambetalieva LB. Juvenile gout in a woman. *Revmatologiia (Mosk)*. 1986;3:67-68.

19. Lugmani RA, Bacon PA, Moots RJ, et al. Birmingham Vasculitis Activity Score (BVAS) in systemic necrotizing vasculitis. *Q J Med*. 1994;87:671-678.

20. Manzi S, Meilahn E, Rairie J, et al. Age-specific incidence rates of myocardial infarction and angina in women with systemic lupus erythematosus: comparison with the Framingham study. *Am J Epidemol*. 1997;145:408-415.

21. Pile K, Kennedy L. *Problem Solving in Rheumatology*. Oxford: Clinical publishing; 2008.

22. Schmidt KL, ed. Soft tissue rheumatism and overload damage. Diagnosis and treatment. In: *Rheumatology Orthopedics*. Wehr: Ciba-Geigy Verlag; 1994 [German].

23. Stone SJ, Stone JH, eds. *A Clinician's Pearls and Mythos in Rheumatology*. London: Springer Science+Business Media BV; 2009.

24. Schwarz-Eywill M, Friedberg R, Stösslein F, et al. Rheumatoid arthritis at the cervical spine an underestimated problem. *Dtsch Med Wochenschr*. 2005;130:1866-1870 [German].

25. Sturm A, Zidek W. *Differential Diagnosis of Internal Medicine*. New York: Georg Thieme Verlag; 2003 [German].

26. Taylor RB. *Difficult Diagnosis*. Philadelphia: W.B. Saunders; 1985.

27. Wollina U, Hansel G, Koch A, et al. Tumor necrosis factor-alpha inhibitor- induced psoriasis or psoriasiform exanthemata: first 120 cases from the literature including a series of six new patients. *Am J Clin Dermatol*. 2008;9:1-14.

Index